Health Coaching Tips and Case Studies

Health Coaching Tips and Case Studies

To Improve Your Coaching Skills

Leila Finn

A big shout out to my colleagues - and especially to the students I have been so privileged to work with - you are powerful change agents dedicated to improving people's lives! Thank you!

Table of Contents

Preface

Finding health coaching is one of the best things that ever happened to me. It taught me how to help other people become empowered in their own self-care. It also taught me how to better empower myself.

I am a health coach and a health coach instructor. When I teach health coaching, students finish the first day realizing that health coaching is not what they thought it was - and finish the last day realizing the life-changing skill it truly is. I have always been interested in how people can create change, and that's what health coaching does; it helps people envision and create the change they want to improve their lives. It provides an opportunity for people to challenge their assumptions about what they can and cannot do. Through coaching, clients learn how to envision what is possible and discover pathways to make that vision a reality.

Health coaching changes lives!

I began my coaching career over ten years ago at the YMCA. Like so many coaches inspired by their own health journey, I wanted to help others with diabetes. I had great success managing type two diabetes and wanted to help others do the same. I was running and enjoying long-distance cycling, and my doctor suggested I get a personal trainer certification. I did, and while I had personal experience and book knowledge, I needed practical experience to help other people reap the benefits of regular physical activity. I volunteered at my local YMCA, and soon after, I was hired to be a wellness coach.

. The wellness coach training at the YMCA was limited (this was also before any national certification), but our YMCA wellness coaches helped many people who otherwise would not have access to health or wellness coaching. The Y is also a charity, and many people who can not otherwise afford to join a gym (or pay for coaching) can join the YMCA through their scholarship program. I love that!

It was while I was at the Y, working as a wellness coach, that I learned about the health coach training program at Duke Integrative Medicine. I remember it well - I was listening to "The People's Pharmacy" on the radio, and they were interviewing Tracy Gaudet, executive director of Duke Integrative Medicine, about their health coaching program. I was so excited - I thought, "that is what I am trying to do!" I immediately enrolled, completed the health coaching foundation course with cohort 4, and immediately after joined Duke's inaugural integrative health coach certification training program, becoming one of the first health coaches certified by Duke Integrative Medicine.

The training I received at Duke gave me a strong foundation. I used my training as a wellness coach at the YMCA. It made me a better lifestyle coach in the Diabetes Prevention Program. Through the Georgia Division of Aging, I worked as a lay leader and master trainer for the Stanford Chronic Disease and Diabetes Self Management Programs, helping to provide programs and training in North Georgia. While not coaching per se, the Stanford programs (now offered through the independent Self Management Resource Center) are infused with coaching theory, and I could see why they were designed the way they were. Working at a national company, coaching patients referred by their health insurance programs, allowed me to engage with clients from all over the country with a broad range of health concerns.

I love teaching, and I was fortunate to be asked to help develop the health coach certificate program at Emory Continuing Education and taught there for seven years. I was an instructor at Georgetown Continuing Education's Health coach certificate program, and I've mentored at the University of Arizona's Center for Integrative Medicine health coach certification program.

I have seen and heard lots of good coaching — and lots of not so good coaching. I have seen health coach training that is very good — and health coach training that lacks depth and sufficient mentoring. As an instructor and mentor, I have seen the common mistakes new coaches often make and have learned what can help them avoid those mistakes and become better, more skillful coaches.

Here I want to share with you what I have learned and offer you practical health coaching tips on how to improve your coaching and avoid common coaching mistakes. I will present case studies based on real coaching experience and walk you through coaching strategy, highlight common pitfalls, and show you how to avoid falling into them.

Whether a novice to coaching or a returning pro looking for a refresher, I hope this serves you well!

Introduction

I wrote this book because I want to offer something that I have not seen: a book with coaching tips with case studies modeled on real-life coaching to illustrate health coaching techniques and strategy.

In these pages, I will give you practical health coaching tips on how to improve your coaching and avoid common coaching mistakes. I will present case studies and walk you through coaching strategy, highlighting common pitfalls, and how to avoid them.

If you are reading this, chances are you already know a lot about health coaching. Perhaps you are a new coach or a veteran health coach looking for ways to continue to hone your craft. That said, health coaching is a new profession, and even with a national board certification now in place, there are still some differing views on what health coaches should and should not do, and how coaches employ specific skills. To ensure that we have a common understanding, let me briefly share my description of what health coaches do.

I will start with what health coaching is not. Health coaching is not giving advice. Health coaches don't tell people what to do, and we don't try to convince clients to take action. We do not educate clients or give them ideas on how to reach their goals. We don't make plans or suggest what clients should or should not do. We don't try to inspire clients to act though our own enthusiasm.

I suspect you know this. And you probably know that telling people what to do or encouraging them to act when they are not ready does not work!

Most of us come to health coaching because we want to help people be well. Many of us have gone through our own health challenges, or we are the ones others come to for advice. But what you discover when you become a health coach is that health coaching is really about helping people find their best way forward.

Health coaching is part of a broader paradigm shift in health care, focusing on patient-centered care.[1] Health coaching is also part of the movement to transform health care from a reactive model that treats people once they are already sick, to a proactive model, focusing more on prevention and what keeps people well.

This is important for several reasons. Much of what makes us ill can be avoided or mitigated. Screenings for disease (to catch conditions early) and vaccines (to prevent illness) are critical. But the most powerful - and cheapest - way we can prevent disease and enjoy good health is by changing our behavior.

In 1900 the leading causes of death were pneumonia, tuberculosis, diarrhea, and heart disease, three being infectious diseases.[2] Today the leading causes of death are heart disease, stroke, chronic lower respiratory diseases, and cancer — conditions that can be treated

---

[1] Muammer and Aldahmash (2018) write : "...by bringing patient-centered health care to the forefront, the patient is no longer a passive recipient of healthcare services and the concepts of patient engagement and empowerment have gained ground since they embolden the role of patients to proactively participate in self-care practices especially in this age of chronic disease upsurge"

[2] The CDC also notes "The 19th century shift in population from country to city that accompanied industrialization and immigration led to overcrowding in poor housing served by inadequate or nonexistent public water supplies and waste-disposal systems. These conditions resulted in repeated outbreaks of cholera, dysentery, TB, typhoid fever, influenza, yellow fever, and malaria."

medically and, more importantly, can be prevented and sometimes reversed by lifestyle change. If you scroll though the Centers for Disease Control and Prevention (CDC) website for what you can do to prevent heart disease, stroke, respiratory disease and cancer the recommendations are consistently the same; to choose healthy foods and drinks, keep a healthy weight, get regular physical activity, and not smoke. [3]

So if it's so easy to prevent disease and premature death, why don't we eat better, move more, and lose weight? I'm willing to bet all of us have all been told by a caring healthcare provider at one time or another to make a change, to lose weight, stop smoking, drink less, start an exercise program, and eat fewer sweets or fast food - and then we don't do it.

It's expert advice - good advice! So why don't we do it?

The American College of Sports Medicine's "Exercise is Medicine" program even has prescription pads for providers to use to "prescribe" exercise.[4] But prescribing lifestyle change does not work. Telling people to make a change, even trying to scare people into making change, does not work.

In the medical world, not doing what you are told is called "non-compliance". Two terms here really illustrate the issue: prescribed and non-compliant. A medical expert prescribes a course of action,

---

[3] Our lifestyle is shortening life expectancy - "researchers found U.S. life expectancy had been increasing for several decades, rising from 69.9 years in 1959 to 78.9 years in 2014. However, the researchers found improvements in life expectancy began to slow down in the 1980s, then leveled off and started to reverse after 2014. According to the researchers, U.S. life expectancy declined for three consecutive years, falling from 78.9 years in 2014 to 78.6 years in 2017." Advisory Board Daily Briefing, December 2, 2019

[4] https://www.exerciseismedicine.org

and if the patient fails to follow the expert's advice, he or she is judged 'non-compliant'. As a result, both the medical practitioner and the patient are frustrated, and both feel stuck. It is neither the patient nor the medical practitioner's fault - but it is a symptom of our reactive medical model that needs revision.

It is simply not enough for a medical expert to tell a patient what to do, and there are so many reasons a person may not do 'what the doctor ordered'. Patients may disagree with their health care providers about a diagnosis or prescription. Costs may be prohibitive. And even with the best of intentions, following advice to make behavior changes to improve health is hard. Moreover, many health care providers are given neither the time nor the skills to have an effective discussion with their patients about why they struggle to change behavior.

For medical care to be effective, we have to know why people aren't doing what they need to improve their health. We need to know what is getting in the way? And to have a productive discussion that helps resolve barriers, there has to be a true collaboration between the health care provider and the patient. Our traditional health care model is a top-down, expert-driven, disease reactive approach. Even with a shift towards patient-centered care, health care providers don't have the time to coach their patients.

A proactive, collaborative, patient-centered healthcare model requires a new approach with a new kind of expert who can support people in making the types of lifestyle changes we know can make people well and keep them well. That is how health coaching came to be. The health coach is the new professional whose sole responsibility is to help people figure out what they need to be well and how to do what they need to be well in a way that works for them.

It is, instead, a bottom-up approach. Health coaching believes fundamentally in the client's wisdom - that each of us has the knowledge and ability to figure out what we need and how we can successfully achieve our goals. Health coaches trust that our clients can find their way - and that they are the experts. Our job is to help our clients find the path that works for them - to let our clients show us where they need to go and how to get there.

When people can tap into what is personally exciting and important about what they want to change, they will be more likely to act. And if people can create a plan for some first steps that they feel are doable, they are more likely to succeed. With success, people build greater confidence - and more success.

Health coaching is a partnership that works because clients are not pushed towards a goal or action that feels unrealistic or out of reach. Let's look more at how this partnership works and how health coaches help clients without telling them what to do.

Charting the Coaching Process

There is a theoretical and practical foundation for health coaching and a fundamental health coaching process that all professional health coaches should recognize and follow. However, different training programs, instructors, and health coach manuals lend their own style and language to describe the coaching process and sometimes differ on what they may include in their curriculum.

It will be easier going forward if we have a shared description of the coaching process and a common set of terms to use later for the tips and strategies I want to share.

Setting the Foundation of Health Coaching

Health coaching follows decades of research in health care and social science. Health coaching itself is also profoundly practical. To be good at health coaching, it is crucial to understand both what you are doing and why. To illustrate the why and the how of health coaching, I propose four foundational pillars of health coaching: Motivational Interviewing, The Transtheoretical Model of Change, positive psychology, and mindfulness.

Motivational Interviewing

"Motivational Interviewing is a collaborative, goal-oriented style of communication with particular attention to the language of change. It is designed to strengthen personal motivation for and commitment to a specific goal by eliciting and exploring the person's own reasons for change within an atmosphere of acceptance and compassion." Miller & Rollnick 2013

Motivational Interviewing evolved from insights clinical psychologist William Miller had on the ability of people to create change when a conversation between therapist and client had specific qualities: that the conversation was client-centered, based in empathy with respect for the client's point of view, and that it focused on the client making his or her own argument for change. [5]

In the 1980s, Miller was working on a treatment for alcohol problems. At the time, behavioral and clinical approaches encouraged confronting people about their alcohol use. Miller saw that confronting clients created resistance. Telling people why they are wrong to continue certain behaviors (drinking, substance abuse) did not work, but effectively communicating empathy and allowing the client to articulate their own reasons for change did work.

He also found that even brief interventions provoke change. In a 1981 study, Miller divided clients seeking help with drinking into two groups. One group was assigned to a counselor for ten weeks of behavior therapy. The second group was given a self-help book with similar material, scheduled for a follow-up meeting ten weeks later. and encouraged to see what they could do on their own during the intervening weeks. The results were startling. The self-help 'control' group did as well as the group meeting with therapists! Miller

---

[5] Miller also found that the ability of a counselor to show empathy correlated to client outcomes. The better a counselor is at listening, understanding, and accurately reflecting what a client says, the more successful the treatment is. (Miller, Taylor and West 1980)

repeated the study several times, once with two more groups who were put on a waiting list and told only to return in ten weeks. These people did not change their drinking habits. And again, those who had the help of therapists and those who were given a self-help book and encouraged to 'see what they could do' did equally well. The people who did not change had done what they were told: to wait.[6]

While teasing out what made self changers as successful as those meeting with counselors, Miller went on sabbatical in Norway. There Miller was asked to demonstrate his counseling style to newly trained therapists. The Norwegians roll played clients and asked Miller questions about why he chose to reflect one thing a client said over another. What was going through his head? What was his decision-making process? This was a turning point and Miller started thinking about how he was navigating the counseling session in a way that encouraged the client to make the argument for change. Miller shared his insights in a paper he sent colleagues and he was encouraged to publish his thoughts. "A Model of Motivational Interviewing", appeared in the British journal Behavioural Psychotherapy in 1983.

In 1989 Miller met Stephen Rollnick, who had been using Miller's Motivational Interviewing (MI) model in healthcare in Great Britain. Thus began a long partnership. In 1992 they published their book Motivational Interviewing: Preparing People to Change Addictive Behavior. Since then, many studies and trials have demonstrated the effectiveness of motivational interviewing in helping people create change not only in substance abuse and health care but in many different settings. There is also now more insight about motivational interviewing and what works and does not. The third edition of their 1992 book, Motivational Interviewing: Helping People Change, further illustrates the knowledge built on over three decades of research and practice with MI.

---

[6] Miller and Harris 1990

Because of its client-centered approach, fundamental respect for the client's point of view, and ability to allow clients to envision and articulate their reasons for change, Motivational Interviewing is central to health coaching. It gives us a powerful and practical way to talk to people about change - and it tells us why it works. If you have completed a health coach training program (especially one that is NBC-HWC approved)[7], you will have learned MI principles, though you may be unfamiliar with MI terminology.

Motivational Interviewing practitioners:

1)   Meet clients with empathy and respect. This helps create a safe environment for clients and reflects the collaborative and non-judgmental nature of MI. The expectation is that given the opportunity, the client will find their way to a solution.

2)   Highlight discrepancies between the client's current behavior and their values. Rollnick and Miller describe people's inability to act for change as ambivalence. As clients develop a picture of what they want, as opposed to what they are doing, they begin to want change. [8]

3)   Don't argue! Arguing with a client or trying to confront them about a belief or behavior erodes trust. You don't have to agree with your client. You do need to meet your client where he or she is - MI gives you the tools to do that.

---

[7] The National Board for Health & Wellness Coaching (NBHWC), https://nbhwc.org

[8] An easy example is a double-sided reflection - a coach might say (based on what the client has shared and not on the coach's opinion): "reading the newspaper is important but stressful, and you think reading a novel would bring a better start to your day" or "going to a gym is not something you want to do, on the other hand, you see getting some more activity in could help you better manage your diabetes".

4)   Support self-efficacy. Clients believe they can make a change when they think they can do it. We want to acknowledge success AND help clients create action plans where they feel very confident they can succeed.

In sum, Motivational Interviewing believes in the individual's wisdom and integrity, and that change is possible when the argument for change comes from the client and not the professional "expert." People do not change unhealthy habits because they are told to change - or because they know the habits are unhealthy. They change because they want to AND because they see a path whereby they can have success.

It is important to note that MI is not a way to trick people into making change. Instead, it is based on the fundamental belief that each of us has the knowledge and ability to help ourselves. When using MI, we are facilitators - assisting others to uncover how they can use what they already have to create what they want. In the latest edition of their book, Motivational Interviewing: Helping People Change, Rollnick and Miller felt it was important to be even more explicit about MI's intent. MI could, for instance, be exploited as a technique to try and sell something to someone. To be abundantly clear, Rollnick and Miller define the four central components of MI's underlying spirit.

Partnership - MI is done for and with another person

Acceptance - Citing the work of psychologist Carl Rogers, Miller and Rollnick describe four aspects of acceptance. Recognizing the *absolute worth* of every human being. *Affirming* people's strengths and effort. *Accurate empathy*, seeking to understand another person's perspective. And *autonomy*, exercising a fundamental respect for each person's freedom and capability to choose.

Compassion - To actively promote and prioritize the other person's needs and welfare.

Evocation - "Evoking what is already present, not installing what is missing."[9] In other words, MI seeks to find the answers the other person already has within them.

Embarking on a coaching journey with a client is like traveling to a land where you might have a compass, but only the client holds the map. Your expertise as a health coach, with fluency in Motivational Interviewing, will allow you to help your client navigate how to get to where he or she ultimately wants to go - but only your client knows the path to get there!

To navigate the collaborative conversation that is Motivational Interviewing, you need to actively listen to your client, turning off your own expectations, interpretations, and judgments, approaching the client with an open mind. This is powerful stuff - rarely do people get to talk with someone who is genuinely listening, without judgment, and without sharing an opinion about what to do. Only with an open mind - and an open heart - can you truly listen to what your client is saying and hear what he or she needs.

There are four critical MI skills: Open questions, Affirmations, Reflective listening, and Summaries.

Try watching the news broadcast and see if you hear any open questions. You don't hear many - they are mostly close-ended, like "do you think Mr. Smith said the right thing?", or "is the price of milk going up?". They are questions that seek to direct the interview. It is also why politicians rarely answer close-ended questions directly with a yes or no! An open question (or an open-ended question) seeks more, "What do you think about what Mr. Smith said?" or "How do you think the price of milk will be affected?". Instead of "do you", "are you" or "is it" ask how, or what, where or when.

In MI, and health coaching, you want to use more open questions than close questions, and you want to use more reflections than open questions.

---

[9] Miller and Rollnick 2013, p 24

Open questions expand the conversation. In health coaching, they will be questions about value, action, and to find focus.

What would be different if you had a regular exercise routine?

Where would you like to see yourself in a year?

How long do you want to walk?

When you are making that choice - what could help you remember what makes this so important?

What do you think is the best place to focus today?

Which of these areas would you like us to address today?

Affirmations, reflective listening, and summaries are all types of reflections. Reflections are statements of what the client has told you. They should not recap everything the client has just said, but rather highlight the most important things the client has shared. An affirmation, recognizing a client's strengths or success, is also a type of reflection.

You want to use your ability to take care of others to take care of yourself.

You've used creativity to find solutions to other challenging problems.

You want to feel better about yourself.

You see the possibilities, now you want to figure out how to get there.

Reflections do a few things. People don't always hear what they say. Reflecting allows the client to hear what they have told you. This can be very powerful, helping your client gain greater insight. Reflections also confirm you are listening and whether you understand what your client is telling you.

Open questions allow you and your client to explore the landscape. You begin to see what is on the map. Reflections help make sure you stay on the right road. They are the easiest way to make sure the client leads you and not the other way around. If you find yourself lost in your coaching, guessing where to go, try reflecting!

By listening to our client's point of view, using open questions and reflections to explore what is important and valuable about change, we tap into what is personally exciting about making change and what will inspire the person to act. Motivational interviewing lends us a way to navigate the map to find out what the client needs, what's important about making change, and how to start to take action.

Fluency in Motivational Interviewing is essential to skillful coaching. Fluency in MI comes from not just understanding what MI does and how, but with lots of practice. The case studies in this book will demonstrate how different types of open questions and reflections work in health coaching sessions. [10]

Now let's turn to our next pillar, the Transtheoretical Model of Change.

---

[10] I have noticed that while health coach training programs use Motivational Interviewing (MI) skills they are not always explicit about what MI is, specific about MI what skills are being taught and may or may not use MI language to describe those skills.

Transtheoretical Model of Change

In the late 1970s, James Prochaska and Carlos DiClemente were looking at how effective different forms of therapy were in helping people make changes in behavior. They concluded that the therapies had similar outcomes and that the therapeutical models had more to say about why people don't change than how they can change. Since the therapies differed little in how effective they were Prochaska and DiClemente shifted their focus to how people succeeded in making change - whether they were successful changing on their own or with a therapist's aid.

Like Miller, Prochaska and DiClemente's research started with people struggling with addiction. While the path to how people came to addiction differed, the road to recovery was the same[11]: all successful change-makers went through a similar process. This process is described as six stages.

As with Motivational Interviewing, what Prochaska and DiClimente learned about how people create change has been studied by many and applies to any context where someone seeks to change a habit.

Transtheoretical Model of Change and Health Coaching

The great majority of health coach clients are thinking about change. They often feel stuck, not able to act. The Transtheoretical model presents a six-stage process by which people transition from accepting the status quo to creating new behavioral norms. Recognizing where a client is in the change process will help you know what kinds of questions and reflections to use and where to focus in the coaching process.

---

[11] Prochaska and DiClemente 1983, Prochaska, DiClemente and Norcross 1992, Prochaska & Velicer, 1997

The six stages of the Transtheoretical Model of Change are:

Pre-contemplation: The client is not ready for change and not thinking about making a change. This person is content with the status quo.

Contemplation: The client is thinking about change and how it might look. This person often feels stuck and uncertain. This is also often the person who has acted in the past and then failed - lost weight and gained it back, quit smoking, and started again.

Preparation: The client is getting ready to make a change and will take action soon. He or she has a plan and is getting ready.

Action: The client is acting, and making changes. It takes thought and planning, but the action is getting done.

Maintenance: The client has been successfully acting and making change for several months.

Termination: The client has succeeded in maintaining change. It is now a habit and routine.

One fundamental tenet in the transtheoretical model is essential to good coaching: a person will not succeed when they are not ready to act. You cannot will yourself into success - "just do it" does not work. When a coach encourages a client to act on a goal that is out of reach, we fail our client. Encouraging people to act before they are ready is why so many diet and exercise programs fail. Wellness programs are usually geared for those ready to take action - not for those who are just thinking about what they could do or working through how they might make it happen. To be effective, health coaches need to recognize where a client is on the change continuum.

While the stages appear linear, the path to change is rarely a straight line. Someone can stay in contemplation, thinking about what they might do, for a very long time, act, and then fail to continue acting, relapsing to contemplation. We see this all the time. I'm sure we can all come up with examples of failing to create a new habit or of falling out of one. New Year's resolutions last for a few weeks or months, and then old habits take over. As coaches, our job is to help our clients better navigate the change process, creating a path forward that works for them.

The great majority of your clients will be in contemplation or preparation, and often uncertain about taking the next step. They feel stuck, questioning why they are unable to act. By helping clients pair their values with action steps they feel confident they can do, health coaches help clients find a way forward. As clients achieve their goals, their self-confidence grows. Success builds upon success. Ultimately the contemplator charts a course that works for them, planning what they can do, acting to meet their goals and create new habits.

Positivity and Health Coaching

Our third pillar of health coaching is positive psychology.

Just as MI seeks to elicit the benefits of change, finding what is intrinsically motivating for each client, health coaching is most successful when clients can build positive goals. This goes hand in hand with the stages of change - acting on something you want is more accessible than acting on something you think you should do (but don't necessarily want to do). Even more intriguing is that positivity and optimism foster creativity, allowing clients to see possibilities about how they might begin to make a change.

Historically, like medicine, psychology was based on a disease model. It sought to understand, diagnose, and treat mental illness. Following World War Two, Abraham Maslow, Carl Rogers and Erich Fromm developed humanistic psychology. (William Miller often refers to his humanist training and conjuring what Carl Rogers would do.)

19

Maslow wrote:

"The science of psychology has been far more successful on the negative than on the positive side; it has revealed to us much about man's shortcomings, his illnesses, his sins, but little about his potentialities, his virtues, his achievable aspirations, or his full psychological height. It is as if psychology had voluntarily restricted itself to only half its rightful jurisdiction, and that the darker, meaner half."

Founders of positive psychology include Martin Seligman and Mihaly Czikszentmihalyi. Their paper, in the February 2000 edition of the journal American Psychologist, "Positive Psychology, An Introduction", defines the need for the field of positive psychology, arguing the need for psychology to focus on what makes people well. They advocate psychology study why some people are more optimistic, happier, and more resilient than others and develop ways to help everyone be happier and more fulfilled. Other prominent figures in positive psychology include Christopher Peterson and Barbara Fredrickson.

Peterson writes:

"Positive psychology is the scientific study of what makes life most worth living. It is a call for psychological science and practice to be as concerned with strength as with weakness; as interested in building the best things in life as in repairing the worst; and as concerned with making the lives of normal people fulfilling as with healing pathology."

Barbara Fredrickson posits that the negative has greater power to direct our emotions and thoughts than the positive, and suggests a ratio of three positives to counter each negative. The math may or may not be fuzzy, but the point is that negativity can easily pull us down. She also posits that positivity allows us to "broaden and build" - to see beyond the negative and exercise creativity, build community, and better thrive.

20

Being positive or optimistic does not mean being Pollyanna. It's not that there is nothing negative, or that some negativity isn't helpful - there are times it is righteous to be angry and appropriate to be sad - but our ability to work through difficult times is easier when we are open to what might be possible. Even in the most difficult circumstances, there is almost always something that can help relieve suffering.

One of the most powerful things about positive psychology is that it shows that we can do concrete things to be happier and more positive. We are empowered to shut off gratuitous sources of negativity and are shown we can intentionally foster sources of positivity and happiness. Focusing on positivity and happiness does not mean denying or avoiding the negative (or sad). We all experience negative, hurtful and sad events, but people who have a more positive outlook rebound from adverse events more quickly. Positivity builds resilience.

Health coaching posits that our clients have the knowledge and wisdom to find their way to achieve their goals - we want our clients to build upon their strengths and celebrate success, be kind to themselves when something doesn't work, and use creative problem solving to find a better way to take that next step. Too often, clients have a narrative about what they can and cannot do. Then when they have trouble taking the next step, they see failure - and quit. Much of the negativity in our everyday lives does not need to command our focus. Health coaching helps clients discover where the negative is keeping them from living their values.

In MI speak, statements that express a preference for change is change talk. As health coaches, we want to listen for and reflect our client's change talk - highlighting what clients say that is positive and valuable about what they want to achieve. The positive, what we value and enjoy, is what inspires. By reflecting value, and asking questions that open the possibility for thought and reflection about what is possible, we help our clients "broaden and build."

Clients are also more successful when they have positive action plans - when it's something they can do instead of something they need to avoid. In her book The Willpower Instinct, Kelly McGonigal writes that when we identify something as dangerous, we look for it. It's instinct - we watch out for what might get us! For example, if I decide I will not eat sweets I will keep scanning for sweets. I'll remind myself, "I can't eat sweets." As McGonigal explains, there are limits to how far willpower can take us, and if I am constantly reminding myself I can't eat sweets, I will eventually give in and eat sweets.

My goal can still be "not to eat sweets" - but my action plan should focus instead on what I can do, not what I can't do. Let's say, I know I will eat sweets in the middle of the afternoon at work, and when I stay up late on the weekend. My positive action plan that focuses on what I can do would be to go outside for ten minutes or watch a funny video instead of wandering into the break room where I will find something sweet. Then for the weekend, I'll keep some healthy snacks I like in the refrigerator. This positive action plan shifts the focus to what I can do instead of what I shouldn't do. Our case studies will further illustrate eliciting change talk and the construction of positive SMART goals and action plans.

Because what is negative has a stronger hold than the positive, we can easily get stuck in the negative muck - stuck in self-doubt and negative self-talk. It's like train tracks in the brain. "There I go doing that again," "I'll never lose weight," "I was so stupid," "why do I say things like that?", "nothing is going my way." It's so easy to jump on board the negativity train! And the more often we jump on board the negativity train, greasing the negative train tracks, the quicker the train goes to its destination.

You start the day in a bad mood, and then nothing goes your way. Traffic is bad. You can't possibly have time for lunch. Too many people are asking too much of you. Your stress builds. But if we can learn to notice when we jump on that negative track, we can intentionally change the dialogue. We can switch trains, begin to grease the positive track, and allow the negative tracks to rust with time and practice. The more we notice, stopping the negativity reflex and looking for the positive, the negative tracks rust, and the positive tracks are easier to ride.

To switch tracks, we have to be intentional and mindful - noticing, and then replacing, the negative: "maybe I can go outside for ten minutes and pick up a sandwich for lunch, the break will make me feel better", "I'm doing well with my food choices", "I'm going to talk with my family about needing some downtime, and maybe we could bring back pizza night so I don't have to cook".

For example, a client says, "walking helps me clear my mind, I'm calmer when I get home, I'm better with my children and spouse, I can think more clearly, I solve problems while exercising." There's a lot of value in that statement - a lot of change talk. Reflect! By reflecting back the positive, the client hears it again.

Reflections highlighting value (the positive) could be:

"It makes everything better"

"Walking gives you clarity"

"Being able to go for a walk gives you so much"

The client will most likely respond to your reflection with more change talk — or you can ask an open question to evoke more change talk.

So imagine if instead of highlighting the positive, you focus on what isn't working:

"But you are too busy right now to walk"

And your client responds, "yes work gets in the way" and "I'm too tired in the morning and home too late at night". If you respond with a reflection that highlights the negative - "it's just really difficult right now" or "you're struggling with where you can find time to walk" - you are likely to elicit more of what isn't working (sustain talk). It's easy to get caught up in what's getting in the way. The key is to strike a balance between acknowledging real barriers and keeping the conversation open to what can work.

23

Focusing on what isn't working deflates the conversation and brings the coaching down - I see this a lot with new coaching or when coaches are rusty. As health coaches we want to take a positive approach because recognizing and building upon our strengths and likes lifts us and allows us to see possibilities. Looking for and acknowledging what is good opens our eyes to more of what is good. Likewise looking for what is wrong or negative has us seeing more of what is bad. If you were to continue to reflect what doesn't work or what gets in the way the negative will drive the coaching session into a downward spiral.

Instead follow with a more positive reflection: "on the one hand time is short, on the other hand if you could get some walking in all kinds of benefits would follow", or you could try something a little more neutral, "you are wondering how you might fit in some walking". These positive reflections, reflections that focus on value and open possibility, help move the coaching forward and encourage the client to think about how they might be able to take steps towards their goal.

To put the negative that does not serve us aside and replace it with more positivity, we need to be mindful. It's easy to go down a negative track but to back out and change direction, we have to notice. Let's now look at our fourth pillar: Mindfulness.

Mindfulness

Jon Kabat-Zinn offers this definition of mindfulness:

"Mindfulness is awareness that arises through paying attention, on purpose, in the present moment, non-judgementally."

We worry about yesterday or plan for tomorrow and often fly through our day following routine. We multitask. We distract ourselves with our phones and have greater access to news and entertainment than ever before. All of this 'noise' can keep us from filtering what is relevant and important. We have to be mindful of what we are doing and thinking when seeking to alter routine and create change. Paying attention, on purpose, in the present moment, non-judgmentally, disengages the noise and puts the break on mindless routine, inviting you to notice the here and now.

"Non-judgementally" dovetails well with positivity and the creativity of 'broaden and build'. If we consider a situation non-judgmentally, we can see more possibilities.

When we don't judge:

We can be as kind to ourselves as we are to other people.

We can look at a problem as a puzzle to be solved, not a failure to be endured.

We can break down a big goal into more manageable bite-size pieces.

I'll lend a personal example. Several years ago, I broke my toe, and I gained fifteen or twenty pounds. I had some complications, and it was several months before I could get back to my run/walk routine that I relied on to keep my weight down. I had to buy new clothes, and I could see the weight stubbornly steady on the scale. But I had an advantage, I am a health coach, and I'd successfully lost weight before. The first thing I did was stop weighing myself. I told my doctor not to tell me what I weighed. I put away clothes that did not fit. I saw a new podiatrist and began going to physical therapy for my plantar fasciitis. I made some dietary tweaks: I remembered I use to follow Mark Bittman's "vegan till six," limiting meat and dairy until evening (this morphed into mostly vegetarian).

It took a while to lose the weight and get back to my exercise routine, but speed was not the point; progress was. Weighing myself had been telling me I failed - when I stopped weighing, I stopped that negative feedback. (I cannot take credit - I got the idea from a conference presentation by a dietician). Likewise, easily grabbing clothes that fit me made me feel good. Seeing a different podiatrist presented me with new treatment options (PT), and eating less meat was something I had wanted to get back to - and was something I knew I could achieve. Are there other things I could have done? Yes. I could have counted calories, gone to the pool, or spin class, and I've done that before and with success, but those felt like chores.

Being mindful and not judging is also something we want to model for our clients. When clients fail to meet a goal, we want them to see it not as a defeat but as a source of information that we can build upon. Making change is about vision, creativity, and problem solving - not judging or blaming. We want clients to notice what they want for themselves and bring awareness to what helps and what gets in the way. Mindfulness is integral to the coaching process for both client and coach.

As a health coach, you are juggling many things - following the client, remembering what they have told you, offering concise reflections, and open questions that lead to more discovery. You are managing your reactions and thoughts and keeping your mind from wandering. You may have other distractions you need to mitigate. Practicing mindfulness helps coaches be present and focused on their clients. As a coach, mindfulness will help you better listen to your client by turning down inner chatter. Practicing mindfulness will make you a better health coach.

Practicing Mindfulness

Inspired by Buddhist style meditation, Jon Kabat-Zinn initially developed the Mindfulness-Based Stress Reduction (MBSR) program at Massachusetts General Hospital to help people suffering from chronic disease. Forty years later, mindfulness meditation has entered the mainstream, and many studies, including technologies like functional MRIs, have measured the benefits of meditation and how it can help everyone.

Meditation changes the brain - functional MRIs have measured structural changes to the brain and show how meditation activates areas of the brain such as self-regulation and problem solving, as well as structural changes in the regions involved in learning, memory and regulating emotion and empathy. There is measurable change even with novice meditators - scans of the brains of participants taking an eight week MBSR workshop, before and after program completion, showed changes in the brain's gray matter. [12]

Practicing mindfulness meditation has many benefits and will improve your ability to be present and aware. Today there are many resources to help people get started with meditation. MBSR classes are available in person or online. Jon Kabat-Zinn has youtube videos, and there are many guided meditations, workbooks, and community-based meditation classes or groups. I like to have multiple resources (especially inexpensive or free) on hand for clients in case they express interest. I've included some in the appendix.

There are other ways to exercise that mindfulness muscle: mind-body exercises such as a progressive muscle relaxation, body scan, or by purposefully bringing attention to the present moment while sitting, walking, or eating.

Other ways to practice mindfulness[13]

As you start a new task, take time to notice and be aware of the present moment.

Take "time out", notice how you are in the moment.

Take a mental vacation, imagining a place you enjoy to get away.

---

[12] Boccia, Piccardi and Guariglia 2015, Marsh 2011

[13] See the appendix for more on mindfulness exercises

Purposefully take a few deeps breathes.

Many health coaching and wellness programs incorporate mindfulness - body scans, guided meditations, and breathing exercises. Practicing these yourself will help you be better versed in describing them to your clients.

The Coaching Process

Our four pillars present the theoretical and philosophical foundation of health coaching. They are the source for both the why and how of health coaching. Motivational Interviewing informs us on how to engage and talk with our clients. The Transtheoretical Model of Change lends us a way to chart the change process and reminds us to identify where our clients are ready to act. Positive psychology tells us that we can achieve better mental, emotional, and physical health by building on our strengths, and mindfulness helps us to be present and aware.

Thus, we come to health coaching with a particular spirit and intent. We are present and focused on where the client will lead us, using our abilities to identify value and vision (change talk) to help our clients find a path towards achieving their health vision.

Now let's turn to what happens during a health coaching session. We will begin by looking at the four processes of Motivational Interviewing, and then build upon that. The four MI processes are *engaging, focusing, evoking, and planning*.

We **engage**, meeting the client and establishing the coaching relationship.

Introducing yourself as a health coach, greeting the client, establishing rapport, and build trust. We are continuing to engage throughout the coaching process.

We establish the **focus** of the coaching session.

A client schedules a session with a health coach, wanting to discuss a particular health concern. The coaching session may be a follow up from a doctor's visit about a specific health problem, or scheduled through a workplace wellness program because the employee has a chronic health condition. The topic may or may not be obvious. The focus of the session can also shift.

For example: A client initially wanting to cook more at home decides establishing a regular exercise routine would be a better and more attainable goal to begin to lose weight. Or a client referred for help with her diabetes wants to focus on reducing her stress and remembering her medication. We want to listen to what is important to the client and where the client sees action as possible.

Evoke what is intrinsically valuable about making change.

Exploring with the client what is valuable about making change - what will be gained by having a regular exercise routine or less stress. What will be different? What will be better?!

We listen for change talk - things the client says that points towards change. We also listen for sustain talk - things the client says that reflects the status quo or what would be different with change. Our mission is to reflect and evoke change talk; this is the client's own argument for change.

Planning what action to take.

Defining what steps the client will take towards achieving their goal. What the client will do next should be both accessible and well defined.

Miller and Rollnick describe these as four processes, rather than phases or stages, to better describe the MI session's fluidity. The

29

same is true in health coaching. While you are setting the tenor for the coaching relationship at the beginning of the coaching session, you will be engaging with the client throughout the coaching session. While you will want to establish the focus of the coaching session early, the focus can shift as your client considers other goals or courses of action. Evoking what is valuable and intrinsically motivating about making change is primarily done as you establish focus and subsequently discuss what the client wants before shifting to planning. However, evoking can continue while planning. A summary of the client's plan might, for example, include a reflection about positive benefits the client anticipates experiencing with the planned action. And while planning will usually take place in the latter half of the session, follow up sessions will often begin by reviewing what happened after the last session - how was the plan, what happened?!

The sequence, however, does matter. New coaches are quick to rush to action, assuming the focus is set and the client ready to act. *You want to cook more at home! What will you cook? You want to exercise more! When will you go to the gym?* It is crucial to remember clients usually come to health coaching not because they are ready to act, but because they are stuck. If you skip past evoking to planning, and force action, the client will fail. A good rule of thumb is to spend half your time in a coaching session establishing focus and uncovering and exploring value (evoke), and half of the session identifying what action the client wants to take (planning), what is do-able, how it will happen, what might get in the way, and if any workarounds are needed to better ensure success.

To recap, the coaching process entails:

Meeting the client - Establishing the coaching relationship.

Finding the topic or focus of the session - What does the client want to talk about? What are their health goals?

Explore value - What is important and valuable about making this change (which is what will motivate the client).

Helping the client define a plan of action - Establishing what action is doable now, what the client wants to do next, and how. The client must be confident they can succeed. We want to meet our clients where they are ready to act — not push them to something they express they should do but are not confident of success.

What precisely will the client be doing between now and the next session? What is the SMART goal? What might get in the way? What can make the plan stronger or easier?

We have looked at the basic coaching process and touched on the evidence-based scholarship and skills that form the foundation of health coaching. Our case studies will further demonstrate the coaching process and how all of these come into play. Now let's look at why an integrative approach to defining good health is helpful to health coaching.

Health Coaching: An Integrative Approach

The World Health Organization defines health as "a state of complete physical, mental and social well-being and not merely the absence of disease or infirmity".

An integrative approach to health encompasses the whole person and recognizes that many factors coalesce in defining good health. Health problems and their solutions are multifaceted, and an integrative approach better allows us to touch on all the moving parts. An integrative approach recognizes that our health goals do not reside in silos. Like diabetes, heart disease, or pain, a chronic condition will affect more than one part of our lives.

Likewise, one action can have multiple benefits. If stress and frustration at work contribute to a person's high blood pressure, taking a pill may help but won't solve the problem at work. Finding ways to reduce or better cope with stress at work might help lower the need for medication. An integrative approach also helps us look at our health with a bigger lens, and helps our clients consider all the parts that interrelate to create good health.

The Wheel of Health

A helpful tool to discuss health and its moving parts is a "wheel of health" or "wellness wheel." A Google search for "wheel of health" provides many examples of health or wellness wheels, usually a circle with pie wedges identifying different health categories: movement and exercise, food and nutrition, relationships, environment, and mindful awareness. Some wheels include additional areas, like spirituality, finances, mind-body connection, sleep, meaningful work, occupation, or career. Rather than wedges I envision spokes on a wheel that interlock to bring strength to the whole.

The wheel of health is a great tool to expand the coaching conversation. It's a canvas for clients to describe their vision of good health and help them see where they might want to act. I've created a wheel of health for this book. I am giving our wheel eight spokes: physical activity, rest and relaxation, food and nutrition, finance, spirituality, occupation/fulfilling work, relationships, and physical environment.[14]

Wheel of Health

Physical activity : Exercise, daily movement, stretching, strength building, endurance, balance, and mobility.

Rest and relaxation : Good sleep, 'down time', or doing something just because it is relaxing and fun. It might mean getting away and going on vacation.

Food and nutrition: Healthy eating, access to fresh foods, having the cooking skills to make meals at home, and meeting nutritional needs.

Finance: Financial security, financial planning. Having the money you need for shelter, food, transportation, education, savings, relaxation, and travel.

---

[14] There is a wheel of health worksheet in the appendix

33

Spirituality: Spiritual fulfillment, faith, connectedness to something other or greater than one's self - mindful awareness, and meditation often go here too.

Occupation/fulfilling work: Paid or volunteer work, career, hobbies. Work that provides intellectual stimulation and satisfaction.

Relationships: Family, friends, community, relating to others.

Physical environment: A safe and comfortable home, neighborhood and surrounding community, access to transportation and other needs, as well as nature.

As we look at the areas that we assigned to each spoke of our health wheel, we can quickly see how these spokes work together. Food and nutrition, for example, often involve relationships. Not everyone at home wants to eat the same foods. Occupation and physical environment come into play - colleagues at work put out candy bowls, or the break room has doughnuts or cake. Work travel makes healthy food choices difficult. These may be multiple challenges — but they also present multiple opportunities to act.

Your client decides to focus first on breakfast and lunch - the meals that don't involve family - before trying to get the family together to create a menu everyone can enjoy. Work travel requires a range of strategies to eat well, from researching restaurant options on the road and carrying healthy snacks, to a plan to counter the temptation of snacks and sweets at meetings.

A client concerned about getting enough sleep looks at the spokes finance and rest and relaxation and shares that needing to work long hours or multiple jobs interferes with sleep and downtime. Thinking about what might help, she decides a short meditation before bed could help her get to sleep more quickly, and that planning leftovers for dinner (food and nutrition) a few days a week would save time cooking and allow for some downtime.[15]

Clients usually come to us with a specific problem or goal. The wheel of health allows us to focus on the topic the client initially presents, and offers the opportunity to explore what else might be important. A client comes to lose weight; he considers the health wheel and decides the most accessible place to start (where he is most confident of success) is in rest and relaxation. Getting to bed earlier will help with snacking, and he has heard that getting enough sleep will help with weight loss. And he feels more confident about getting to bed earlier than he does about embarking on a diet plan.

An integrative approach also allows clients to step back and take in the big picture of what they want for themselves. It's something we don't often do - and it can lead to new insight and different ways of thinking about health. We are used to thinking about health as "not being sick" but we don't often think about what makes us well or more healthy. And in thinking about health, we don't often think about what makes us happy, but happiness is an essential part of good health.

Here are some more examples of goals that involve multiple spokes of the wheel of health:

"I need to work from home so I can be there when my child comes home from school. I will also need to create a dedicated space for my work - I somehow need to carve out office space!".

Here we see occupation, relationships and environment (and probably finance).

"I need to find a dietitian to help me with my diabetes but I am on medicaid and I can't find someone I can get to easily on the bus".

---

[15] These solutions work because they are conceived by our clients to meet the unique challenges they are experiencing.

Here we have food, finance, and physical environment.

"I want to cook more vegetarian meals at home but no one else in the family wants to try new meal ideas. I don't want to cook two or three different meals!"

Food, relationships, and maybe rest and relaxation if the client wants to keep cooking to a minimum to have some downtime in the evening.

Health goals are multifaceted and complex. It would be easy to pick out one piece of the puzzle and go into "fix it" mode. That's what people do all the time. In response, someone trying to help might say:

Where do you want your office?

You need to take a longer bus ride.

What extra vegetables do you want to make for yourself?

An integrative approach reminds us to look further, and listen for *the different moving parts.*

Having an office might be less important to the client than making sure he makes the best use of the time he has alone to get his work done. Then he can better engage with his daughter when she comes home from school.

Instead of a longer bus ride where there may or may not be a dietitian, the client may decide a better solution is to see what other programs might be available nearby, talking with her physician, or doing some research online. She might already have another idea, deciding instead to focus on eating less take out food.

Making extra vegetables for herself may be one solution, but it ignores the importance of cooking less. Other people are often obstacles, and this client might instead prefer to focus on her other meals and decides she can make more progress with breakfast and lunch and tackle dinner later.

An integrative approach helps both coach and client uncover and explore both what's going on and what solutions can work. As a coach you can use a descriptive tool like the wheel of health or just use the concept in your coaching sessions. Either way, it helps us remember to look at the whole picture.

Looking at our wheel of health, what areas do you see where you would like to make some changes? There is a wheel of health worksheet in the appendix.

Case study: Considering the Wheel of Health

Gloria is seeing a health coach as part of her participation in a workplace wellness program. Her coach introduces her to the wheel of health, broadening their discussion about Gloria's goals and aspirations. Here, the coach uses the wheel of health to open up the discussion to explore how the client envisions health and well-being. What does she want for herself? And what are her immediate and long term health goals?

Coach: Hi, Gloria! Thank you for coming today. It's good to meet you.

Gloria: Good to meet you too.

Coach: We talked on the phone some about health coaching, and I know you had some concerns about privacy. I just want to assure you that nothing said here will be shared with anyone else, including your employer.

Gloria: Thank you - I was worried about that.

Coach: You share only what you want to share, and whatever you say here stays here.

Gloria: Ok, thank you.

Coach: You signed up for the weight loss program, and you mentioned on the phone that you want to lose sixty pounds.

Gloria: Yes.

Coach: And we can absolutely talk about what will help you meet your weight loss goals. I'd also like to ask you about your health goals overall, and I have a nifty tool I can share with you if that's ok.

Gloria: Yes, that's fine

Coach: (Getting ready to show the wheel of health) What does good health mean to you, what does it look like?

Gloria: Having more energy, getting my blood pressure down, it is one reason I want to lose weight. My mother had a stroke. I don't want to be a burden to anybody - I'm almost sixty, and I want to be able to do what I want to do. I want to look good too!

Coach: The word that comes to mind is vibrant!

Gloria: Vibrant - yes! I have things to do and places to go!

Coach: You have plans.

Gloria: I retire in a few years. I want to travel and move to a smaller house. Spend more time with my grandchildren.

Coach: You have some exciting changes coming soon.

Gloria: Yes!

Coach: (Shows picture of the wheel of health) Awesome. I'm interested to see what you think of this because it relates to a few things you've just said. This is the wheel of health - it helps us look at all the different parts of our lives that inter-relate to create good health. Good health is about more than not being ill - and someone can have a diagnosis or disease and be well in other ways. You've already touched on a few areas, retiring - and travel, maybe that's rest and relaxation. That could be occupation and fulfilling work, not working at your job but engaging in things that are intellectually and emotionally fulfilling. Environment, moving, and having a smaller home. Family - relationships. Taking a moment to look at these, what else pops out?

Gloria: Finance is good. Physical activity - I used to be more active. That's part of why I've gained this weight.

Coach: You think more physical activity would help you lose weight.

Gloria: And keep me strong, so I can do what I want.

Coach: And be vibrant!

Gloria: Exactly!

Coach: And you said you used to be more physically active, tell me more about that.

Gloria: I used to live by the beach, and I loved to ride my bike along the boardwalk. I'd walk on the beach. I love the ocean, but I moved for my job and to be closer to my children.

Coach: You had a nice routine

Gloria: I did, but it's nice here too, and I like being near my children and I have a lot of friends here.

Coach: So it was a good move. You just need to find a routine that works for you here.

Gloria: Yes, because I used to do those things, I suppose I could bike on the path — or walk. I guess I'm not sure what I would want to commit to.

Coach: Not quite sure what adding back more physical activity will look like, but something you see yourself doing.

Gloria: Definitely!

Coach: Looking at the wheel, what else stands out?

Gloria: Well, food, of course. I've signed up for the weight loss program, and so far, I like their approach. It's not about dieting per se, no counting calories, but more about being mindful about your choices. I'm trying to be patient - it's going to take a while.

Coach: You know it's going to take some time, and you want to stay on track

Gloria: Yes. Right now, we are focusing on mindful eating. Not eating too fast or being distracted - like I usually eat lunch at my desk while I'm on the computer. That also means I order out whatever the rest of the office orders, which is not good. So I'm going to the break room and paying attention to what I'm eating and eating more slowly. And it's true, doing that I don't eat as much. Now I need to pack my lunch - I'll save money that way too.

Coach: Practicing mindful eating has already changed how you eat!

Gloria: It has. And I'm trying to practice it more at home. Even if I eat while watching TV, I pay attention to my food, paying attention to the taste, and eating more slowly.

Coach: Doing this at home now too - sounds like it's working for you.

Gloria: It is. And if I want ice cream or something sweet, I wait ten minutes. If I still want the ice cream, I get some but usually, I forget. So it's not too hard.

40

Coach: Wow, that's great. So food and weight loss - and mindful eating - sitting in "food and nutrition," anything else that's important or valuable about food?

Gloria: Nutrition - that's part of making some better choices. And the salt - the doctor told me less salt could help lower my blood pressure, and I don't want to have to take more medication. I'm hoping that if I can lose weight, eat less salt, and get some regular exercise, I can lower my medication. I don't know if I can get off of it but at least not have to take more. As I said, I don't want to have a stroke like my mother.

Coach: Right! And you have a clear vision of what you need to do.

Gloria: I know what I need to do. I just got to do it all!

Coach: And that's what we can do here - figure out how you can approach these goals in a way that you can be successful.

Gloria: That would be great.

Coach: We've touched on a lot of things in the wheel - what about spirituality? What are your thoughts about that?

Gloria: I grew up going to church. I didn't take my children - I couldn't find a church I felt comfortable with. And that's fine. I have God in my heart.

Coach: Feeling good about where you are in spirituality

Gloria: Yes

Coach: And how about rest and relaxation?

Gloria: Well, retiring! I can go to the beach more often, and I want to take some big trips. And just not work so many hours. I'll probably do some part-time work or volunteer - I don't see myself sitting around - but on my schedule.

41

Coach: What do rest and relaxation mean before retirement?

Gloria: Good question! Not bringing work home - that's the big one.

Coach: Leaving work at work.

Gloria: That's it!

Coach: For rest and relaxation, long term, retiring, being your own boss! And short term leaving work at work.

Gloria: Yes!

Coach: Looking at the other parts of the wheel of health, you are already making some changes around food and nutrition. You're taking the weight loss program and have some specific goals around food choices and taking lunch to work. You mentioned lowering salt could help with your blood pressure. And that's a big concern - you want to do all you can to stay healthy, lower your risk of a stroke. Getting some regular physical activity is a part of that as well, and you're not quite sure what that looks like yet, but something you've done before and want to work back in. You have a good sense of spirituality, and it sounds like you have an excellent plan financially as you are getting ready for retirement. That dovetails with the environment - you'd like to downsize, and I think I heard you say you'd like to get back to the beach more often?

Gloria: Yes, I do.

Coach: Important to be near friends and family here but getting that beach fix! And in the short term, rest and relaxation mean leaving work at work.

Gloria: Yes, work at work, and less stress. I've enjoyed this - I wasn't sure what we were going to do!

Coach: Good! And next time, we can look at some of these goals and what you want to approach next, whether it's taking lunch to work, how to reduce your salt, exercise, leaving work at work. It's really about breaking down these bigger goals into do-able, bite-size pieces in a way that you can have success.

Gloria: That sounds great - thank you.

Coach: Thank you, Gloria! I look forward to seeing you in our next session.

Case study: An integrative approach (not using the wheel)

Let's look at another case study, this time using an integrative approach but not explicitly referencing the wheel of health. This time it's about listening for and following up on the parts of the wheel - the parts of our lives that inter-relate, describing an integrative approach to health. This time our client is Denise. She has pulmonary fibrosis and is on disability and has been referred to a health coach by her health insurance company. We will jump in after Denise has met her coach, and they have gone through an introduction packet on health coaching.

Coach: I know you've been referred to health coaching because of the problems you have with your breathing. Thinking about your overall health a year from now - where would you like to see yourself?

Denise: I want to be doing more. I'm home all the time, and I don't see many people, I see my husband and my youngest son, but I'm pretty limited in what I can do.

Coach: Doing more, getting out more.

Denise: Getting out more but not relying on my husband so much. I have been volunteering with a project at the archives doing some translation work, and that's been very interesting, plus I can do as little or as much as I want. It's good to have something to do -

something you know where you can feel like you are contributing. But around the house, I can't do much, and it's hard to go out.

Coach: You've found work that you enjoy - and there's more that you'd like to be able to do. Tell me more about that.

Denise: I'd like to be able to make dinner sometimes - Steve usually cooks, and I'd like to be able to help. I'm trying to eat more too. I'm having a hard time eating enough.

Coach: So two things, you'd like to pitch in more with dinner, and you want to see how you can eat more.

Denise: Yes, and when I think about in a year or more, I think about how I don't want to be frail. I'd like to be able to walk to the park - it's just a few blocks away. It would be wonderful to be able to take an afternoon stroll.

Coach: Getting your strength up - more endurance.

Denise: Yes, and the people at rehab say I should be able to do all of that - with the rehab and keeping my weight up. I want to do more for myself, like I've been going to rehab, and I'd like to be able to get there on my own. My husband or my son takes me now.

Coach: You want to be more self-sufficient!

Denise: I do! And having the archive work has been great- it doesn't get me out of the house, but it is interesting it gives me something of my own to talk about.

Coach: The archive work sounds great - that's so cool you can do that.

Denise: I'm so glad I found it, and I love history and am fluent in Spanish. I translate letters and journals. I feel like I'm meeting these people from the past.

Coach: That's awesome - and it sounds fulfilling. You've mentioned several other things that are important to you too , eating more and building your strength and stamina - and you are already going to rehab. You want to get to where you can walk to the park, getting out of the house more - seeing people, helping more with dinner, and generally being more self-sufficient and independent.

You can see how this summary quickly touches on four or five parts of the wheel of health - fulfilling work, relationships, physical activity, food and nutrition, and physical environment. Notice too a common thread is being self-sufficient. We know that all of the wheel's areas or spokes inter-relate. No one health issue is divorced from the other areas of our clients' lives. My case studies reflect the shared struggles and aspirations of many real clients, and this one includes experiences of clients dealing with disabling lung diseases. Common threads in many cases also include conflicts with family, financial strain, and other people not understanding what they were going through. As you allow the client to lead you, listen for areas of the wheel. An integrative approach helps you 'open up' the coaching - for example let's say Denise begins by saying she needs to eat more but has little appetite. If the coach acknowledges the concern - "you'd like to be able to eat more" - but keeps the door open - "what else would you like to be able to do?" - the client will come back with more. The focus may still be on eating and appetite, but it might turn out to be something else. If instead, Denise's coach fixates on appetite, exploring value (what would be better if she could eat more), and transitions to SMART goals and action plans (how can she eat more?) too quickly, the coach will miss the opportunity to see what else is there - what else might the client want? And, by focusing only on appetite, the coach makes a common coaching mistake by running with the first goal the client expresses - I call this "jumping on the first train". We want to see what other goals or concerns the client might have - what other trains might come by! This is especially important if the goal is very challenging -and the client's confidence is low. Denise might want to focus solely on how she can eat more, but she might prefer to talk first about getting her family to stop bugging her about how little she eats, or how she can get to rehab on her own. Let's continue with our case study and see what does happen!

Coach: Tell me more about being stronger and more self-sufficient.

Denise: Like I said, getting to rehab on my own - and I think I can do that now. I just need to figure out how the mobility bus works.

Coach: Going to rehab on your own - what else would you like to see, say in the next six months?

Denise: I'd like to make dinner. Go out to lunch - that would be nice. Just have enough strength and energy I can enjoy going out.

Coach: Where you don't have to worry about having enough energy.

Denise: Yes. It's so tiresome. I have friends invite me to go out to their house, even offering to pick me up and take me home - but I'd be embarrassed if I needed help to get back to the car or if I fell asleep.

Coach: You'd like to feel confident about a visit with your friends.

Denise: That would be great - and I know I'll get there. I just have to remember how far I've come already.

Coach: You've already done a lot of work. Work towards getting better, being stronger and more independent, and getting out more and doing more things that you used to do.

Denise: Yes - feel more like my old self.

Coach: And rehab comes to mind - working your way back up.

Denise: Yes!

Coach: And you said something earlier - that the work at the archives gives you something of your own to talk about. Can you tell me more about that?

Denise: Oh, that is the hardest thing - it's like my illness is my job, and there's nothing exciting or interesting to talk about. I mean, my family and friends are great, but I want to be able to tell them about what I've done - I mean, it isn't all about me, but you want to contribute something to the conversation.

Coach: A coloring book comes to mind - It's like some of the colors has been washed away, and you want to fill it back in

Denise: Yes, I want to color in more things I can do, more places I can go.

Coach: A big piece of that is getting stronger.

Denise: Yes - and I do know I can get stronger. I just have to keep going to rehab and work on eating more. I'm very good about doing exercises at home too.

Coach: Awesome - you're doing the exercise you need to get done.

Denise: Yes, and I see progress, and the therapists are very encouraging.

Coach: Tell me more about eating.

Denise: I just don't have much appetite. I'm better about eating dinner - it helps that I'm not eating alone, but it's more problematic during the day.

Coach: What would you like to see yourself eating?

Denise: I'm pretty good at eating some cream of wheat or a bagel at breakfast. Sometimes I snack on some nuts. I like pistachios. Lunch is more challenging - its better if I don't have to make much. I tried those shakes in a can, but it was gross. Half a sandwich is good - I try to have some meat and cheese for protein, and it tastes good. I should have a snack in the afternoon, and I usually skip that.

Coach: Eating more between breakfast and dinner.

Denise: Yes - more lunch, an afternoon snack.

Coach: And it sounds like some foods are more enticing than others - like NOT shakes!

Denise: Yeah - no, shakes! It's texture and some things just don't taste good. Like ham and cheese is good but not peanut butter. Tunafish salad is good. I think I like salt! Oh, and I should drink more water.

Coach: So water too.

Denise: Yes, and I have a big water mug I carry around. I have been better about that.

Coach: You are working on staying hydrated.

Denise: Yes.

Coach: So what we want to do is take those bigger goals - like having enough strength to go to out, to walk to the park, see friends - do more! And make a plan for how you build towards that goal week to week. Thinking about the next two weeks, what seems like a do-able goal in terms of building your strength?

Denise: It's funny - I was just thinking I could make a sandwich at lunch, and instead of making just half a sandwich, I could make a whole sandwich - eat half at lunch and a half later in the afternoon.

Coach: Your afternoon snack would already be made!

Denise: I could have tea time! And hot tea would be good too.

Coach: A half sandwich and a cup of tea - when is tea time?

Denise: Four is good - that's when I like to take a break anyway.

Coach: How confident do you feel that that will work?

Denise: You know I'm pretty confident - I want to try that.

Coach: Awesome! Anything else that might help?

Denise: Just that I have sandwich stuff - but that's not a problem. Yeah, I think that might work.

Coach: Anything else around strength that you want to do this next two weeks?

Denise: No - really just doing the rehab and exercises.

Coach: You also mentioned wanting to go to rehab on your own, helping with dinner - or making dinner. Would you like to look at those - or something else you'd like to have as a goal for these next two weeks?

Denise: I like the idea of making dinner together, but I'm not sure how much Steve wants me messing with his prep, but I could keep him company. I'll talk with him about it - it could be some nice together time. I don't think I'm up to making a real dinner yet, but I'm going to suggest we order out on Friday. It's one way I can give him a break.

Coach: Suggesting takeout - and maybe changing that evening dynamic, so you are both in the kitchen.

Denise: Yes - that sounds good.

Coach: And I just want to check in on the rehab - you mentioned looking into the mobility bus

Denise: Yeah, I don't really want to do that. Its a great service, but friends at rehab have told me it takes a lot of time. I should probably figure out how to use Uber, maybe later.

Coach: Ok - so maybe another strategy later. Anything else?

49

Denise: No, I think that's good!

Coach: Great! These next two weeks, when you make lunch, making a whole sandwich, saving the second half to have in the afternoon - around four - tea time! Will you be having a sandwich for every lunch?

Denise: Yes - there might be a day or two when I have leftovers, but a sandwich is easiest.

Coach: You'll have lunch and your tea time snack. You also want to order take out as a way to pitch in and talk with your husband about keeping him company while he is making dinner. What do you think?

Denise: That all sounds good.

Coach: And anything you need to remind you of your goals? For the sandwich, ordering out, or talking with your husband about dinner?

Denise: I should remember, and he'll be home soon. I'll tell him what we talked about.

Coach: So, do you feel like you have a plan?!

Denise: I do!

Finding Focus and Knowing When to Move to Action

A Common Mistake - Taking the First Train

A client comes to their health coach with a problem: health coach and client talk. The client comes up with a plan. Session done! It sounds simple, but we know there is a lot more to it than that, and the problem first presented is not always the most important. Coaches want to take care in establishing the focus of the health coach session, listening for what else might be there.

As a health coach, it is tempting to "jump on the first train" and coach around the first topic the client presents. Better quality coaching happens when the coach takes note of that first train - but takes time to explore the problem and see what else pops up. What other trains might come by? A client wants to eat better, but the real problem isn't the ability to make good choices but access to better choices.

For one client, an obstacle (preventing access) to better food choices might mean that someone else is cooking the family meals, and the client doesn't want to hurt the other person's feelings. For another, it's constant business travel and having to eat out. Other common barriers to healthy eating are cost, the lack of knowledge and cooking skills - not knowing what to eat or how to cook different foods.

Let's look at a case study:

Alice has had a heart attack and has been advised to eat a heart healthy diet. She wants to avoid fast food and eat more vegetables and fish. There are two trains here - fast food and eating more vegetables and fish. We can start by exploring the value of avoiding fast food and the benefits of more vegetables and fish and then shift to how she can implement these goals, or we can step back a moment - and see what other trains might come by!

"Avoiding fast food, incorporating more fish and vegetables - what else would be heart healthy?"

And Alice says reducing her sodium intake - that's why she wants to avoid fast food. It has a lot of salt. She says more fruit and fiber are supposed to be good too. Her doctor gave her a book on heart health, and she likes that it mentioned dark chocolate is heart-healthy - she likes that idea! She would also like to start walking - both for her heart and to lose some weight.

There's a lot of information here - and lots of ideas (trains)! Now we want to see both what Alice considers the most important place to start - and where her confidence lies.

Let's summarize: "Lots of ideas - avoiding fast food to reduce salt, more vegetables, fish, fruit and fiber. You mentioned a book you've been reading with some ideas - like chocolate! And walking," We can stop there and see what else Alice might add - or we can start to hone in and ask, "What feels like the best place to start with these heart-healthy changes?"

Alice could come back with any - or even all - of these options, but she is most likely to go to what she feels most comfortable tackling now. And that's important because we want to her achieve success quickly so she builds confidence to take on harder items. Alice says she wants to finish the book her doctor gave her and then meet with her doctor to discuss a plan. She feels good about avoiding fast food, and while fish is an ok idea, she really only likes salmon and tuna fish, and she's unclear about how much fish or what kind she should eat and if she will like other fish if that's what she has to eat. Alice is ok with more fruit and vegetables - she was even vegetarian for a while when she was younger. Alice is excited to start walking. She used to be more fit, but long hours at the office derailed her, and she wants to turn that around.

Two trains have led to many more - summarizing has helped us (and Alice) figure out where she wants to make her first steps. We've also learned more about where she is most excited (walking), where she feels confident (fruit and veg), and where she has prior experience (vegetarian eating and exercise). Now we can shift to planning, defining a SMART goal, and action plan.

Alice decides she will start walking every day after work. She will also leave work smack at 5:30 - this heart attack has been a wake-up call! Not working late will also help keep her from picking up fast food for dinner. She's going to go through her recipe book to refresh herself on some of her old vegetarian favorite dishes and cook at least three dinners this week - on Saturday, Sunday, and Wednesday. She wants to check out the farmers market Saturday morning to shop for some fresh produce, and she wants to finish the book her doctor gave her. She will finish the book this weekend-she's been taking notes and will make an appointment with her doctor when she has finished, probably within a couple of weeks. She's not sure about the fish - she'll ask the doctor more about it when she has her appointment - or the book might tell her more.

The coach will want to check in - how does she feel about her plan? What is her level of confidence that she can do this? Alice feels great! She's excited to get started, and she is confident she will be successful.

We started with avoiding fast food and eating more fish and vegetables. By not jumping on that first train (or two), we've discovered a lot more about what Alice might do and where she feels confident about taking action. These are positive steps she feels good about, and that build on her strengths and knowledge. Note, eating fish is there, but it's on the tentative side - that's fine. Her goal about the fish - eating salmon once a week - seeing if the book says more, and talking to her doctor - meets her readiness level.

Here's what that exchange might look like:

Coach: So Alice, you're here because you want to have a more heart-healthy diet.

Alice: Yes - I had a heart attack, and I want to eat better and exercise so I can do what I can so I don't go through that again. I want to be healthy.

Coach: You had a real scare! And you want to be proactive.

Alice: Oh yes, so scary.

Coach: Tell me more about being healthy.

Alice: Getting my blood pressure down - and I'm on a statin. I had a stent and my doctor told me I could do a lot by changing my diet and walking every day.

Coach: Some real concrete things you can do.

Alice: Yes. Walking every day - she said that's ok. I like that both for my heart and to lose some weight. And eating more fish, less fast food, and more vegetables.

Coach: Avoiding fast food, incorporating more fish and vegetables - what else would be heart healthy?

Alice: Lowering my sodium - that's why not getting fast food is good. More fruit and fiber is supposed to be good too. And walking! She gave me a book about reversing heart disease.

Coach: What do you think of the book?

Alice: It's very interesting. It recommends some tests that my doctor is doing. It says to eat fish three times a week, a lot of vegetarian dishes - beans, lentils, and nuts. You can have some cheese, but it likes some types of cheese more than others. And it has tips for eating out. It also says to have some dark chocolate every day - I like that!

Coach: A lot of ideas!

Alice: Almost too many ideas!

Coach: A lot to choose from.

Alice: Yes, it's a lot to take in.

Coach: Some concrete things you mentioned - avoiding fast food to reduce salt, more vegetables, fish, fruit, and fiber -chocolate! Walking. What feels like the best place to start with these heart-healthy changes?

Alice: Chocolate! - I'm kidding - I want to finish the book my doctor gave me and meet with her to talk about a plan.

Coach: See what else it says and then talk with your doctor to see what is best for you.

Alice: Exactly, because there is a lot in there.

Coach: It sounds like it is giving you some good ideas.

Alice: Yes.

Coach: What else are you thinking?

Alice: That this was a real wake up call. I'm trying to reduce stress and work less. What was happening was I would work late and then pick up something to eat on my way home from work. I want to leave work smack at 5:30 - then I'll have time to walk.

Coach: Getting home in time for a walk!

Alice: Yes! And time to cook. I like cooking - I just got into a bad habit of trying to wait out traffic by working late. I actually used to be a vegetarian when I was younger and more fit.

Coach: Healthy eating is something that has been important to you.

Alice: Yes.

Coach: And you mentioned chocolate - and fish.

Alice: I'm good with chocolate! Fish not so much- I like some salmon and tuna ok, I may ask my doctor about that when I talk to her.

Coach: Ok! And tell me more about less stress.

Alice: I take on too much - but I can leave work on time. And with some planning, cooking should be pretty straightforward - and it's relaxing. I want to look through some of my old cookbooks - remember some of my favorite dishes.

Coach: Cook to relax! Is that something you'd like to do this next week or two?

Alice: Yes - I can do that.

Coach: Looking at some recipes, coming home early, cooking - paint for me what you'd like the next two weeks to look like.

Alice: I do want to finish that book - I can do that this weekend, but yeah, leaving work at 5:30, I'll be home by 6:15. That gives me time to change and walk for half an hour before settling in for the evening.

Coach: Sounds great. What does dinner look like?

Alice: On Sunday, I've been doing something in the crockpot and then eat leftovers for the next couple of days. If I don't feel like much, I'll make some toast and scrambled eggs. And like last night I bought a roast chicken and had a big salad - I'll probably do that again.

Coach: You've been making more meals at home.

Alice: Yes, I know I'm a better cook than that, though - that's why I want to finish that book and look through more of my old recipes. At least to start getting some more ideas - liven it up!

Coach: Take it up a notch or two!

Alice: Exactly.

Coach: We've been talking about dinner - what about the rest of the day food-wise?

Alice: I don't eat breakfast. I'm happy with just coffee. I order out for lunch a lot, and I have been trying to do better there. There is a deli that delivers to the office, and they have some nice options. The main thing is getting home on time.

Coach: Making sure you leave at 5:30.

Alice: Yes. That's key.

Coach: It's the end of the working day where you really want to focus, is that right?

Alice: Yes. If I can leave by 5:30, I can walk and make dinner.

Coach: You've had some success leaving at 5:30, thinking about this next week, on a scale of one to ten, with ten being very confident and one being not at all confident, how confident are you that you can leave work at 5:30?

Alice: I'm going to say a nine because like I said, this was a real wake-up call, and there no reason I can't leave - it's not like there's anyone else there!

Coach: It's that important.

Alice: Yes.

Coach: And when you get home, going for that walk and making dinner. What does that look like this week after work?

Alice: Come home and change, go for a walk. Then watch the news for a bit and start dinner.

Coach: What do you need to for those dinners? You mentioned you use the crockpot, sometimes do an easy dinner like scrambled eggs, looking for some of your old favorite vegetarian recipes.

Alice: I put together a shopping list on Saturday. Go to the farmers market to see what looks good - and then stop by the grocery store. But yes, I did want to look at those cookbooks. I'll do that before I make my list, pick a few dishes to make for dinner.

Coach: So, checking out recipes, making your list before you go shopping Saturday.

Alice: Yes, I like that.

Coach: Great! And do you need anything for lunch?

Alice: No - not now. I may try taking some leftovers. And I may get some nuts for snacks, but I need to think about that.

Coach: Perfect - and you want to finish the book this weekend and then meet to talk about a plan.

Alice: Yes, I can finish that this weekend too - I don't have much left, and I've been taking notes, so I know what I want to ask.

Coach: So this week, key - leaving work at 5:30! Getting home to walk for thirty minutes, then watching the news and making dinner. You'll pick some recipes ad make your shopping list Saturday - Saturday morning?

Alice: Yes, while I have coffee

Coach: Great - making your list, shopping, and finishing the book.

Alice: Yes.

Coach: How does that feel?

Alice: That feels great! I'm excited.

Coach: Excellent! I am looking forward to hearing about your week next time!

Let's try another:

Marcus has type 2 diabetes. He is a truck driver and has been consistently gaining weight over the past ten years. He does long hauls that limit his ability to exercise as well as his meal options. He wants to lose weight and better control his diabetes.

It would be easy to jump on the first train and go straight to action - "How can you exercise more and make better food choices"? Marcus may reply with some ideas like walking around the truck stop parking lot or packing some sandwiches in a cooler. But, he could also say something like, "If I knew that I wouldn't be here", or

"That's just it - I have to eat where I can park my truck, and the only exercise options I have are to walk around the parking lot". Instead, let's explore what else is important about controlling his diabetes and losing weight.

Let's reflect "These long drives leave you with few options, and you'd like to stop the weight creeping up."

And Marcus says, yes - he wants to stop gaining weight. If he can lose fifty pounds, his doctor thinks he could take a lot less medication. He'd be healthier, feel better, and save money. Marcus says he's been thinking about switching jobs and doing early runs around the city instead of multi-day long hauls, but he enjoys being on the road. His wife is a teacher, and during summer break, she will go with him - that's always a treat! On the other hand, he would be home more if he did local runs.

There's a lot here! We could jump on the job train and talk about how he could find a new job doing local drives - but that would be both going straight to action, and the coach would be deciding where the solution lay (getting another job). Remember, too, Marcus is unsure about giving up the benefits of the long hauls. It is better to explore more - reflecting will keep us close to the client and allow him to lead us to where he wants to go.

We could do a double-sided reflection; "On the one hand, you enjoy the long drives, especially when your wife can join you in the summer, on the other hand, a local job would let you be at home more and give you more options in terms of eating and exercise." That would be ok - but I'd prefer to wait and keep it more open.

Instead, let's try "You already have some ideas."

You can leave it there or ask something like "tell me more." Even better would be to go back to value.

Coach: "You already have some ideas, and whatever you decide job-wise, you want to have a strategy to lose weight, take less medication, and save some money!"

Marcus replies, "I have been thinking about it - if I was home more I'd have more options and it'd probably be easier to lose the weight. But I've been doing this a long time and my wife and me, we kinda have a groove. Our plan has always been for me to quit when she retires. Then we'd get an RV and drive around the country ! And she can retire in a few years. I'd like to keep driving long hauls till then. It's not long to wait and the money is good."

Coach: "You have a real vision of where you want to be in a few years."

Marcus: "Yes. We are even buying an RV soon - start doing some weekend camping trips. I want to lose this weight so I can be healthier and really enjoy retirement."

It's already clear Marcus wants to stay in the job he has - lets reflect, including both value and an opening to start thinking about action, ie how Marcus can lose weight.

Coach: "You and your wife have a really solid plan for what you want as you transition into retirement. The key is figuring out how you can lose weight while you are still doing the long hauls, losing that fifty pounds so you can be healthier and save money. And you mentioned that finding a way to have better meal options and getting in more physical activity would both be ways to lose weight."

Marcus replies: "Yes, exactly. I was thinking about the local runs, but yeah, I don't want to have to find a new job with just a few years left till I quit."

Let's go to action — we have found a lot of value and narrowed in on what and where Marcus wants to act. Let's check.

Coach: "Thinking about how you can fit this into your current routine, adding some healthier food choices, some exercise, what do you see yourself doing?"

Notice that inherent in this question is the assumption Marcus has ideas and that this is possible! A positive approach helps generate solutions. We want to focus on what he can do - not on what he can't do, doing long hauls.

Marcus: "I want to get a fridge for my cab - they are little, but you can keep stuff for sandwiches. I have a small microwave too. I can bring frozen dinners and carry cold cuts for lunch. I used to have a fridge, but it broke, and I just haven't gotten a new one, and I'll admit I like getting out of the truck to eat, but if I eat out less, it will also help me save more money for the RV."

Coach: "Having a fridge will give you a lot more options."

We want to pull out change talk and focus on the positive action - but we don't want to ignore the other value nuggets. *Marcus wants some time out of the truck.* Let's check in on that.

Coach: "It sounds like it's also important to have some time away from the truck, and to eat out was one way to get a break."

We could ask what other ways he could get a break from the truck, but by reflecting, we let Marcus show us where he wants to go.

Marcus: "It is, but it's not good for my middle! It's more important that I eat better and save money. Not eating out will make a big difference. I can get some walking in when I'm waiting for the truck to be loaded or unloaded, and I can do more when I am home."

Let's summarize the plan so far -

Coach: "Getting a fridge for your cab so you can bring your food. And you said you could take a walk when you are waiting at your drop off or pick up points, and there is the opportunity to do more walking when you are home."

Marcus: "Yes - my wife and I like to hike, and I want to get in better shape for more of that, especially once we have the RV. "

Let's go to action - here we have a close-ended question to check-in.

Coach: "That sounds fun. Is the fridge the first step?"

Marcus: "Yes, I'll order it today - I should be able to get it by next week. I'm home for a few days - I'll do some walking in the morning before it gets too hot."

Coach: "Awesome! What days do you want to walk in the morning?"

Marcus: "Oh, I can go out for about an hour every day I'm home."

How confident is Marcus?[16]

Coach: "On a scale for one to ten, one being not confident at all, and ten being very very confident, how confident are you that you can get those walks in and the fridge?"

Marcus: "Oh it's a ten!"

Coach: "Really confident!! And how about the walking when loading and unloading? on a scale from one to ten?"

Marcus: "Maybe more like a seven. It's fine at home - not as sure at the loading dock."

Coach: "So a seven - a little more unsure than you are on the road - what makes it a seven and not a four?"

Marcus: "Because I have a plan - I know what I want to do. I just have to figure out some of the exercise part."

And now we can wrap it up. If you have more time, you can do a SMART goal for the at-home walking, or see if Marcus wants to

---

[16] We will look at how to use the confidence ruler later.

explore more about exercise on the road and any other planning he might need for his meals while traveling.

Value and Intrinsic Motivation

Knowing that change is important and feeling motivated to act to change are two very different things. There is always value in the status quo, even with it doesn't serve our interests.

In Motivational Interviewing, Miller and Rollnick call this *ambivalence*, defining ambivalence as *"The simultaneous presence of competing motivations for and against change"*[17] The Transtheoretical Model of Change labels this state of ambivalence as contemplation. In describing someone in *contemplation*, Prochaska, Norcross, and DiClemente write, *"You know your destination, and even how to get there, but you are not quite ready to go yet. Many people remain stuck in the contemplation stage for a very long time."*[18]

The tipping point between thinking about change and taking action is twofold:

· The person favors change over the status quo.

· The person feels confident they can succeed.

---

[17] 2013, p.405

[18] 2007, p.42

Why people want change and the steps they can take to get there are different for each of us. Health coaches first help clients identify what changes they want and why. What is better with change? What is significant about making this change? By taking time to explore the benefits of change, the coach helps the client develop his or her own argument for change.

Each of us has an individual worldview. Our expectations and interpretations of the world differ based on our life experiences. What I find so powerful about health coaching is its ability to help people challenge assumptions that hold them back. Clients become change agents, discovering how they can create the changes they want.

An effective health coach actively listens to their clients. Active listening means hearing what the other person is telling you. You want to listen without interpreting what you hear and suspending judgment about what the other person should or should not be doing or thinking. It also means being present. In a typical conversation between friends, we think about what we want to say next, adding our opinion or experience, going back and forth with questions, anecdotes, and suggestions. We might debate facts or share a passion. In health coaching, we are turning all of that down, listing without judgment, with an ear towards hearing the client's world view. What is important for her in making a change? What does she want? To eat better, exercise more, quit smoking, change her job, live somewhere else, or better manage chronic disease?

I had a client who wanted to quit smoking. He had lots of reasons for quitting: saving money, having his house and clothes smoke-free, improving his health, but still he couldn't entirely quit. He managed to quit when he realized two things. First, that he could enjoy a beer without a cigarette because while he wanted to quit smoking, he did not want to stop drinking. And secondly, he realized that he would feel stupid if he got sick and died because he couldn't keep himself from giving money to Phillip Morris (by buying cigarettes). There is absolutely no way I could guess that these would ultimately be the motivating factors that enabled him to quit smoking. Only by listening, asking questions that encouraged him to think about what was Important to him about not smoking, and using reflections to highlight what he shared as valuable about making this change, could I create a space where he realized that it was important to him to not feel stupid (and that he thought giving money to Philip Morris for something that he knew could potentially shorten his life) -- and that beer and cigarettes did not have to go together.

As health coaches, we are experts in change, but we are not experts on our clients or their health - they are. When we let them, they will tell us - and themselves:

- What is intrinsically motivating (why they want change over status quo).

- What next steps they can take where they are confident of success.

Evoking intrinsic motivation - exploring value

To tip the scales toward change, the weight of why I want change has to be greater than the comfort of not making change.

To help clients tip the scales and gain the momentum they need to make a change, we need to spend time exploring value - or in MI Speak - evoke intrinsic motivation. We want to take time for our clients to make their own argument for change - ticking off all the reasons why change is good. Successful change happens not because you know you should change but because you want to change. Building a foundation about what is valuable about change allows the client to reflect and solidify the contemplative, ambivalent, 'should' into an actionable 'want'.

Should vs. Want

When people are stuck, thinking about change but unable to act, they are responding to conflicting values.

"I should eat better, but I don't want to give up the foods I like."

"I should cook at home, but I like the convenience of ready to eat meals and take out."

"I should measure my blood sugar, but I don't like what the numbers are telling me."

"I should exercise, but I don't like getting sweaty, and I don't know what to do."

If we simply ask what is important about exercising or eating better, we may get a personal, emotional response but we are also likely to get a response reflecting what the client knows (or has been told) they should do.

"If I ate better and cooked at home, I would lose weight."

"If I tested my blood sugar, I'd know if my medication was working."

We would know the intended result but not the motivation. Knowing that if you exercise and make different food choices, you can lose weight is not inspirational. If it were, we would not have an obesity epidemic!

So instead of starting out with a question like "Tell me what is important about making this change," ask something that will encourage the client to envision what it will be like achieving change:

"Being stronger, fitter, how will your life be different?"

"I could enjoy more activities, and I could continue to live independently, have less pain, and feel more like my old self! I'd look better."

"Losing this weight, what will that mean for you?"

"I would be more confident. I could buy clothes at a regular store, and I could lower my medication and save money, I wouldn't be so hard on myself."

"Achieving this change, what else will be possible?"

"I'd be more likely to date, and I might buy a swimsuit and go to the beach! I'd feel confident enough to look for a better job."

Then reflect the value you've heard. Your client will tell you more about what is important about making change.

It's also powerful for clients to hear what they value spoken by someone else - sometimes clients don't really hear what they say!

When reflecting the value statements, you hear, be concise and try not to use the word "important" or "valuable." Rather reflect what the client has said is important. For example, a client has told you she enjoys shopping. It helps her relax; it's fun, but it costs her a lot of money, and she really needs to start saving more. You can reflect, "you want the joy of shopping without the spending."

Open questions open the door to more value (change talk); reflections highlight the most salient or important thing(s) the client has told you.

"What would be different?"

"How would you feel?"

"Where would you like to be in six months, a year?"

Your client may respond with reasons for why it's easier not to change (sustain talk):

"Getting Uber eats saves time and allows everyone to pick what they want to eat."

"Not exercising means I have more downtime to relax."

"Moving hurts."

Reflect the conflicting values - and give extra weight to what the client wants to change:

"Ordering out has been a way to save time and make everyone happy, and you think it would be healthier for all of you if you had more home-cooked meals."

Ask questions to uncover more value:

"You'd have a little less downtime - what would you gain?"

Meet your client where he or she is:

"You're struggling because moving hurts, and you've been told if you could incorporate more regular exercise, you'd have less pain, and you're not sure how you can start moving more."

When you take the time to explore all that is valuable about change, you will also hear what else is contributing to ambivalence. You are giving your client the time and space to think through what they want. This often leads to the client telling you what other actions might be possible.

Remember to use more reflections than questions - reflections will keep you on track following the client. Practice using reflections, try using three reflections to every question. Summaries can help you when you are unsure where to go. Practice following the thread, listening, and identifying when you start to steer the coaching conversation to what you think is important. I often see students try to guess where the client wants to go - instead, let the client show you. That's the magic of coaching - trust in the process, and your clients will find their path forward.

The focus may shift as you begin coaching. That's ok - if you are uncertain, ask! "You've mentioned several places you'd like to start making some changes - what would you like to focus on today?"

We want to explore value to elicit what is valuable about making change. Don't jump to action without taking time to explore value. Build the foundation for change! Next is planning what action to take but first let's consider the role of the Importance and Confidence Rulers and how they can help us assess focus and readiness to act.

Importance and Confidence Rulers

You can use importance and confidence rulers to gauge where your client is, both in motivation and readiness to act. [19]

The Importance Ruler

Is the topic or focus of the session important to the client? You can use the importance ruler. Ask, "On a scale from one to ten, one

---

[19] The Importance and Confidence Rulers are described in Miller and Rollnick 2013

being not important and ten being very important, how important is [X]?"

The number the client chooses will give you an idea of where the client is in the stages of change. A seven or higher tells you this is important to the client. A very low number suggests it is not important (early contemplation) or not at all important (pre-contemplation) and the client is either uncertain about change or not interested in change.

Your clients will likely be in contemplation. They are coming to you for help precisely because they are stuck! People not thinking about change will be clients who are sent to you by someone else, like someone required to complete a wellness program at work to keep their insurance premium down. You can tell when a client doesn't want to talk about a particular health topic - and the ruler can confirm your instinct! Don't try to push your client ("but your doctor is concerned about...."), instead meet your client where they are: "this isn't something you are worried about, and you're here because your employer sent you", or "You're not so sure it's important, but your doctor thinks you should make some changes." See what comes back, and reflect more.

When this happens, it is especially important to stay in value, allowing the client to lead you to what might be important about that particular topic or goal. Your client will show you whether they want to continue to pursue the original low number topic and if it's a dead-end ("I'm just not going to change what I'm doing") invite your client to share what is something where they would like to see a change.[20] This respects the client and builds trust. And remember, going to another health topic, where the client has more confidence and interest, both allows the client to act on what is important to them and build self-efficacy, making more difficult topics more approachable later.

---

[20] Use the wheel of health!

That said, the great majority of your clients are coming to you because they are contemplating change. They know what they want to change, even if they are stuck. Their response to the importance ruler will be high, a seven, eight, nine or ten! Just remember because something is important, even very important, it does not mean a client is ready to act. This is where health coaches can get into trouble. They take a high importance number as a cue to jump to action. Instead, use the importance ruler to begin to explore value.

"On a scale of one to ten, with one being not at all important, and ten being extremely important, how important is finding a job that will give you more time at home?" Your client responds, "very important - a nine!". Ask "what make it a nine and not a six?" Your client will most likely respond with reasons why being home more is important: "I want to be at my children's school events, I'm missing out on a lot. I'm tired of working so much - I need more downtime." Reflect value! "More family time, more down time." Your reflection about what the client wants will elicit more. Then you can ask, "what does that look like, being home more?", "what does it feel like to work less?"

Notice we asked "what makes it a nine and not a six", encouraging the client to reflect on what makes finding a job that will allow more time at home important. We get change talk. If we asked the opposite, "what makes it a nine and not a ten?" we might get more about what makes this important, but we are more likely to get sustain talk, especially when the numbers are lower.

If we were to ask what might make the importance number higher, "What makes this a six and not an eight?" we might be asking our client to describe something that may not be tangible. "I don't know - I'm just not there." We might highlight ambivalence, "I miss going to school events, but I like traveling, and I make good money which allows us to go on family vacations." As a general rule of thumb, it's best to have the client reflect on what already makes this important rather than encourage reflection on why it's not more important.

73

The Confidence Ruler

The confidence ruler helps assess readiness to act. "On a scale of one to ten, one being not at all confident and ten being very confident, how confident are you that you can accomplish X?"

This helps you and your client assess if the client is ready to start taking action, if the specific action plan is achievable and whether it needs adjusting. For example, your client has been uncertain about getting enough time to tackle a cluttered home office. You have been exploring with your client what makes having this uncluttered, peaceful space at home so important, and the client has painted a picture that she is really excited about. You could just ask, "what steps do you see yourself taking this week towards creating that peaceful, uncluttered workspace?" Or you could use the confidence ruler: "on a scale of one to ten, how confident are you that you can start to take steps towards creating that peaceful, uncluttered workspace?". Both are good questions, but the ruler will give you an indication of how confident the client is she can take steps now. It also provides the opportunity to ask the client to reflect back on why she is confident (why her response is a higher rather than a lower number). There is always some type of action that is accessible - you just have to listen to where your client is ready to take action.

In action we want to do what we generally want to avoid in value. While a client often can't tell you why something isn't more important, your client can often tell you what action is more do-able. Remember, it is important that health coaches help clients create an action plan that meets clients where they are and not push them to set expectations they cannot meet. We want our clients to succeed and build confidence.

"I can't devote a lot of time right now to decluttering, but I could spend ten minutes a day, and that would add up!"

The other place to use the confidence ruler is after your client defines the SMART Goal and Action Plan.[21] Summarize the plan and ask, "On a scale from one to ten, how confident are you this plan will work?". If your client comes in low, you know you need to go back and help your client figure out a plan that is do-able!

A seven or higher generally indicates the client feels confident they can complete the action, a six or below tells you that the client is likely not ready to act. If the response is a low number (one to six) that's your cue to reassess. Did you go too quickly to action, not spending time to explore what makes this change so valuable? Did you listen to what the client actually wants do? Is the scope - or scale - of action too great?

I often see coaches confuse the importance and confidence rulers. Just remember importance goes with value, and confidence goes with action. In contemplation I can believe something is very important yet still be unable to act - my confidence will be low. If you ask me the importance ruler at the end of the session, after devising the SMART Goal and Action Plan, my answer should be high, but that does not assess how confident I am now that I can take action. Importance first, confidence later!

---

[21] SMART Goals and Action Plans are next!

Planning and Taking Action: SMART Goals and Action Plans

People often move from contemplation to planning and action, act for a while, and then fall back into contemplation. We can help our clients better navigate their way from contemplation through action to maintenance by ensuring the action meets the client where they are ready to act. Many wellness initiatives fail because they assume employees or enrollees are ready to act when they are really in contemplation. When you push people to act before they are ready, they are likely to fail - and relapse.

As you transition from evoking into planning, resist the urge to suggest, and instead explore what steps your client feels confident about taking. What your client plans to do should meet where they are in the stages of change. An action might be a step in preparation to act. For example, someone who wants to exercise needs to find a new space for an exercise bike. Another client with a new diagnosis wants to do research before seeking a second opinion, and a third person wants to schedule time to outline a plan.

What the client wants to do may be clear. If not, you can ask, "what action do you see yourself taking these next two weeks?". You can use a summary to reflect what your client has said: "You've mentioned several things you'd like to do within the next six months to improve your health. Remembering to take your medication in the

76

evening, going to body pump, and clearing out space at home, so you have room to workout at home." Then ask: "Where would you like to focus first?"

I've often seen coaches go 'lite' on action. Planning what the client will do is just as important as laying out why the client wants change. Let's look at an example: our client says she wants to focus on making sure she takes her medication every night.

"Lite" would be to end the session there; "Great! You have a plan! The next two weeks you'll take your medication at night!".

Defining a SMART goal:

Better is to define a **SMART** goal. A SMART goal spells out more specifics.

Specific - what action will you take?

Measurable - how long, how much, how often will you take action?

Attainable or achievable - can you accomplish your goal in the timeframe you have set for yourself? There should be a high level of confidence in success.

Relevant - Does your short term goal align with your long term objectives?

Time-based - When will you act?

Example of a SMART goal:

I will take my medication every night, one metformin pill, just before I eat dinner. I am confident I will remember because I will leave my pills in the silverware drawer to remind me. Taking my pill every night will help me better control my diabetes.

This specific: *I will take one metformin pill every night.*

This is measurable: *One pill every night before dinner.*

This is achievable: *I feel confident I can remember, esp. if I put my pill bottle in the silverware drawer.*

This is Relevant: *Remembering to take my metformin every night will help me control my diabetes long term.*

This is time-based: *I will take it every night, before dinner.*

Defining what action the client will take and how is important. When we are trying to do something new or something we have been unable to achieve, we have to create structure to re-enforce action. Notice here, putting the pill bottle in the silverware drawer is key to remembering to take the metformin and makes the goal achievable! If we left it "lite" ("Great! You have a plan! The next two weeks you'll take your medication at night!") our client might not have come up with the idea of putting the metformin in the drawer!

Even better - support the SMART Goal with an Action Plan!

A SMART goal is good - especially if you are short on time, but an action plan spells out the particulars and workarounds for possible obstacles.

The Action Plan

What else will help our client succeed in taking her metformin every night? What might get in the way? When will she put the pill bottle in the drawer, and how will she remember to put it in the drawer?

78

Are there any obstacles? What might get in the way? What would make taking action easier? As we talk further with our client to flesh out the action plan, we find out that she wants to put the pill bottle in the drawer, but she also wants to keep pills in the bathroom because she takes her morning pill when she brushes her teeth in the morning. She decides to put half of her pills in a container in the bathroom. Asked if there anything that might get in the way of her taking her pill before dinner, she responds that there are nights she goes out for dinner. She feels ok about taking the pill in front of her friends, but not if she is out on a date or with people she doesn't know so well, especially at work events. She decides if she is out with people who are not close friends, she can excuse herself to go to the lady's room to wash her hands and take the pill while she is away from the table.

Now we have identified obstacles and workarounds.

Let's summarize the plan - our client will divvy up her metformin into two pill containers, one goes in the bathroom and one in the silverware drawer. There are nights she goes out to dinner or events, and depending on who she is with, she will take her pill at the table or away from the table.

Let's check in on some more detail - "It sounds like having the pills in the drawer is key to remembering them at night -anything you need to remember to take the pill when you go out?". And our client responds she can put a reminder on her phone calendar to put a pill in her purse, and she feels like if she can manage to take the pill in the evening at home for a few weeks, she will remember when she goes out.

I always like to check in on whether my client wants a reminder of her plan - does she want something to remind her of her plan?

Now our client has a SMART Goal and an Action Plan!

Let's do another.

This client says her long-term goal is to be more physically fit, and she would like to be able to ride her bicycle thirty miles like she used to!

To begin to work towards her long term goal, she says she will go to the gym two times a week. Ask, how long will she work out at the gym? What will she do there? What days, and at what time in the day will she go? And how confident does she feel about her plan?

Here is her SMART goal: *"I will go to the gym two times this week and ride the spin bike for 30 minutes. I will do this on Sunday morning, right after breakfast, and on Thursday, on my way home from work. I feel very confident I can do this, and riding the spin bike is a good way to start getting in shape for outdoor rides."*

Now let's make the action plan. What will make the SMART goal easier? What might get in the way? Asking your client to visualize what will happen can help sort out the details and uncover any possible obstacles. Let's ask, "walk me through what will happen Sunday."

"Well, usually I sleep in a bit and have a late breakfast...if I'm going to the gym, I won't want to eat - I can't exercise right after eating. I want to go on Sunday morning because the gym is quiet, and I'm more likely to get a good spin bike. The gym opens at ten so I can still sleep in, get up around 8:30, and have some coffee before I have to get dressed and leave. I'll be done by 11. I guess I can go home and have lunch or pick something up if I want to run some errands. I should probably pack a snack in case I'm hungry."

What about Thursday night?

"I'll need to pack my workout clothes Wednesday night and put them in the car - I think I'll be more likely to go to the gym if I change at work. I'll want an easy dinner that night too since I won't have as much time to cook"

New actions have ripple effects - taking time to go to the gym will take time out of the evening to make dinner. Going to workout in the morning means skipping breakfast. What can make the plan stronger?

"For Sunday, I'll get out my workout clothes Saturday evening, and I'll pack a snack. Having a plan for dinner Thursday would be good - I can make sure I have leftovers from Tuesday or Wednesday"

This is a good time to summarize the goal and check-in with the confidence ruler. Confidence should be high - if not, the plan needs adjusting.

A well defined SMART goal and action plan will help your clients be better prepared and lends the structure needed when making change.

The Need For Structure In Managing Change

Health coaching encourages clients to take time to explore why making change is important to them. The coaching process gives clients space and time to visualize what might be possible and think through what they want. The focus may shift as clients find their footing and realize there are different ways to approach the task at hand. This is what we mean when coaches talk about trusting in the client's wisdom — if we hold that space for the client to consider how and where they want to go, the client will lead us there.

People don't often have the luxury of mulling through a problem with someone who will not offer advice or direction. A skilled coach helps the client focus on what they want and need, frequently leading to a shift in perspective. Creative "fixes" happen when clients have the opportunity to consider other ways of doing (or being). Often big "aha!" moments happen when a client realizes they don't believe a certain narrative or that they have to achieve a goal in a particular way.

But even good change upsets routine. To stay on course, clients need to define what they want and how to get there. A well-defined SMART goal and action plan lend the framework for managing change and provides the structure needed for reordering routine. The SMART goal and action plan is a roadmap you've helped your client create to chart their path towards their goal. Earlier, we likened the coaching process to a compass - if we stay true to the coaching process, our clients will show us what they need to change, and why. The client's map reveals itself and allows us to navigate what a client wants, charting how they can get to their destination.

Case Study: The Domino Effect

Susan wants to get to bed earlier. She wants to get more sleep and go to bed early enough, so it's not hard to get up in the morning. Her coach begins by exploring the benefits of more sleep and then takes time to explore what else impacts Susan's ability to get enough sleep.

Coach: Waking up, feeling rested. Tell me more about getting to bed early and having more sleep.

Susan: I would love to be able to get up without my alarm clock - or at least without hitting the snooze button! If I can get to bed earlier, I can get up on time. Now I hit the snooze button and stay I bed as long as I can and end up rushing to get dressed and out the door to work.

Coach: Getting up easily - feeling rested - and having time to get ready for your day!

Susan: Yes, I'm frequently late to work, and then I end up working later than I like to make up for it. I'd like to be able to sit and enjoy some coffee, pack my lunch, and hit the road a little earlier.

Coach: Imagining this more leisurely morning, waking and feeling rested, what does it look like?

Susan: I wake up rested. I get out of bed right away, and I make some coffee. Read the paper - or maybe a book - just for twenty minutes or so. Put my lunch together, shower, get dressed, and get out the door by 7:30.

Coach: Imagining that morning - how does that feel?

Susan: Awesome!

Coach: On a scale from one to ten, with one being not at all important and ten being very important, where would you put getting to bed earlier so you have enough sleep and feel rested?

Susan: I guess an eight.

Coach: What makes it an eight and not a six?

Susan: My kids are grown and off on their own.

Coach: You're not having to take care of them.

Susan: No. But you know that's how it started. I would make dinner, make sure they were set for the next day and then when they were finally settled, watch some late night TV to wind down. My husband can just go straight to bed — but I need to read or watch some tv first.

Coach: Staying up late was something that developed when you had other responsibilities with your children at home.

Susan: Yes, but I still managed to get to work on time - probably because I had to get the kids out!

Coach: Getting the kids out helped push you out the door - and now you'd like instead to have a more relaxed morning and still get out by 7:30.

Susan: Yes. I don't need to push myself with less sleep.

Coach: Let me see if I can summarize what you've said so far— and tell me if I have this right - while your kids were still at home, you had a lot to do in the evening, making dinner, making sure they had everything they needed for the next day, that they were in bed. Then you could have some downtime - staying up longer, reading or watching tv - and then you could go to sleep. You got up and got out of the house on time because you had to get the kids to school, and that got you out the door too. What you want now is a more peaceful morning and break the habit of staying up late.

Susan: Yes, exactly. I'm addicted to late-night comedy! My husband's in bed by 10:30, he gets up early to go to the gym, but I stay up and watch late-night TV.

Coach: What would you like your evening to look like?

Susan: I think I need to get up at 6:00, so maybe try for 10:30 - maybe 11:00 to start? 10:00 would probably be best to go to bed, but that seems too early. I don't think I'd go to sleep.

Coach: 10:30 feels do-able?

Susan: Mmmmmmm maybe 11:00, 10:30-11:00. I think that's do-able.

Coach: What would it look like, going to bed 10:30-11:00?

Susan: I can't watch my late TV show. Though it's silly - I mean, I could record and watch them anytime! Part of it is I like to stay up to date on political news, and I enjoy the commentary.

Coach: On the one hand, there is a lot of value in watching the late shows. On the other hand, they keep you up later than you'd like.

Susan: You know I can watch them when I get home from work. In fact, a few nights a week, my husband makes dinner now. I usually watch the news then, but I could watch late-night comedy instead. Then I could get to bed on time - read a bit to get me to sleep.

Coach: Get your comedy fix earlier!

Susan: Yes - that would work!

Coach: Watching late-night comedy the nights that your husband makes dinner - instead of the news. What about the other nights?

Susan: I'm not going to worry about Friday and Saturday. We tend to go out one of those nights anyway. I think just focus on work nights. I could watch the days I cook while I'm cooking - or after dinner with my husband.

Coach: You can enjoy watching the shows earlier, and that will allow you to get to bed earlier.

Susan: Yes! I think that will work.

Coach: Can you think of anything that might get in the way?

Susan: I'll need to see how to record or stream the shows, but that should be easy. I can do that this evening.

Coach: Anything else that will help you have that more relaxed morning where you can feel not rushed but still get out by 7:30?

Susan: Having my clothes out. I can do that when I change after I get home from work. I usually go for a walk with the dog before dinner. I can get my clothes out then.

Coach: I'm curious - you mentioned you often stay late at work to make up for getting in late. What about when you get to work on time?

Susan: I can leave on time!

Coach: Another benefit of going to bed earlier.

Susan: Absolutely.

Coach: So, your goal is to get up at 6:00 am, giving you enough time for a nice start to your day, leaving for work by 7:30, getting to work on time. To get enough sleep to wake up at 6:00 am feeling rested you'll go to bed between 10:30 and 11:00, reading a little to get you to sleep. You mentioned putting your clothes out the evening before will help you in the morning. You'll watch your comedy shows earlier in the evening, while your husband cooks or while you are cooking or after dinner, and you will see how to record those this evening so you can have them ready to watch. And a bonus to getting work on time will be getting home earlier!

Susan: Yes. I feel like I have a plan!

Coach: Wonderful - do you need anything to help remember your plan?

Susan: I like the idea of putting my clothes out the night before — I'll put a note in my sneakers, so I remember. Otherwise, all good!

This is a common scenario. Clients want to get up early - often to accomplish another goal, like exercise - and find themselves staying up too late. If we leave the coaching at just getting up early, we will miss the other obstacle - going to bed late. If we focus only on the time to go to bed and don't explore competing factors, the client won't succeed in going to bed early. Common obstacles to going to bed earlier are getting other tasks done, like laundry, cleaning, playing games on the computer, and working. For many, it is valuable alone time , particularly for parents or caregivers. As coaches, we need to be sure to contextualize the goal and listen for competing interests or needs to catch the domino effect!

Navigating Common Health Coaching Challenges

I remember experiencing these challenges, and I see them often when I mentor health coaches. Here are some common coaching challenges, how to recognize them, and how to work your way out!

Not Knowing Where to Go!

You are coaching a client, and you have no idea where to go. A client is stuck, or it's a topic where you have no knowledge or expertise, and you feel lost. This is when the magic of coaching shines through. Trust that the client knows where to go.

Reflections will keep you on track. You can't stray far from your client when you reflect; just remember to use reflections that move the coaching forward by highlighting change talk. You can use a reflection that acknowledges difficulty or sadness but be careful not to use a series of negative reflections. It will elicit more sustain talk and drag the coaching down.

A client is stuck; it could be changing how they eat, exercise, or finding a better job:

Client: I know what I should do, but I just can't seem to do it.

Coach: You can't quite get over the starting line.

Client: I have no time for it.

A client had surgery - it doesn't matter what kind of surgery or procedure:

Coach: This was not an outcome you expected.

Client: No, it's so uncomfortable.

Coach: This is a surprise.

Client: It is.

Our instinct is to help when we see a client stuck, especially if they are suffering. We want to point to answers, and when we can't, it's easy to feel out of depth. Not knowing where to go, coaches often use close-ended questions - trying to find an answer.

Can you go on the weekend?

Is something else easier?

Maybe you could talk to the surgeon?

Is there a patient support group?

The coach is fishing - casting out the line to see if they can catch a bite. If you find yourself stuck, guessing where you should go, stop and reflect.

"On the one hand, you feel stuck. On the other hand, doing this would mean a lot to you. There would be new possibilities."

You could stop there, see what the client says, or follow with a value question, "What would be different if you could do this?" or "How would it feel to get past the starting line?"

Let's look at the client who had surgery. They had an unexpected outcome; a skin graft was needed for reconstruction surgery, amputation makes sitting uncomfortable, cancer treatment leads to hair loss.

You can reflect "sitting with ease." You can leave it there and see what your client says, or ask an open question to what else the client might want: "what else?".

You can try going bigger, "You had the surgery (or treatment) - huge step - and now that you are on the other side of it, seeing that you have some unexpected consequences. What do you think would help you most as you find your feet?". Let the client tell you where they need to go.

When stuck and trying to find where to go, coaches sometimes "jump on the first train" and go too quickly to action. "You want to figure out how to sit more comfortably," or "finding how best to cope with your hair loss." These clients might have that action in mind, but let's first go big before narrowing into SMART goals and action plans. There is likely a lot more there.

Where's the train?

I remember waiting for the train. I was a new coach and had a client who had chronic pain and wanted to lose weight. It was painful to exercise, and she said she did not want to go on a diet. I didn't know what to do! So I let her talk. Eventually - I figured - the train would show up, and she'd show me where to go, or she would eventually come up with something she could do. We did eventually find an actionable goal that could bring her one step closer to losing weight, but the session took much longer than it should have.

Encouraging a client to talk (and talk and talk) in hopes that you will hear a train is natural but inefficient and risky. Instead, follow the coaching process. This client was stuck and had some significant obstacles. She was trying to act (exercise) and failing (because she hurt).

Instead of waiting for the train, explore value. Use the importance ruler. Ask a vision question, where would she like to see herself in six months or a year? What would be possible, what doors would open, what would be different? Your client will respond with what is valuable about exercising or losing weight; they will respond with more change talk. Keep possibilities for action open. When a client is given time to flesh out why a goal is important, they will be more likely to develop ideas about what to do. Keep an open mind about action - a client may begin by saying they want to exercise and not diet, but let's see where they go as we navigate the coaching process.

After exploring value, check-in. If exercising is too difficult right now, what might be do-able? Our client has young children and hates to see food wasted. She nibbles on the children's leftovers as she cleans up the dinner table. She resolves not to eat the leftovers but instead decides to subscribe to the composting service she's been contemplating - and compost what the children leave on their plates. She also shares that she works late at night on the computer - it's the only quiet time she has to catch up on her work. She snacks to keep her self up. She decides she will brush her teeth after dinner, knowing that she won't eat anything else once she has brushed her teeth. She can drink water while she is on the computer, and drinking more water is something else she has wanted to do. Use the confidence ruler - what does she think? She's a ten!

Health coaching encourages clients to see other ways of doing. Trust the coaching process, and you won't get stuck.

The Need to Know More

Another thing coaches will do when they feel stuck is to ask the client for more information, feeling that they could figure out where to go if they knew more. This is especially tempting when a client presents a topic about which the coach has no knowledge. It is tempting to ask the client to explain or give more information.

For example, a coach with little knowledge about diabetes has a client, Joe, who says he needs to test his blood glucose level before he works-out. He says he often forgets his meter at home or brings it to the gym but forgets to take it out and test before getting on the elliptical or going to spin class. Feeling stuck, the coach asks, "how does the meter work?" or "what will testing your glucose tell you?". Now the client is educating the coach, and the coaching process is stalled. We don't want to put clients in the role of educating the coach. It puts the focus on the needs of the coach and pulls attention away from the client.

Instead, follow the coaching process. Look for value - "If you can remember to use your meter, how will your workout be then?", or use the importance ruler "on a scale from 1 to 10 how important is it to remember to check your blood glucose?", or even "and what if you don't check it?". All of these elicit value and help set up the shift to identifying barriers and defining a SMART goal and action plan.

Joe tells his coach he has gotten lazy. He used to test a lot more, but his A1Cs have been good, and he's enjoyed a break from testing. An affirmation about his A1c would be good. "That's great - that took a lot of work!". Then the coach can explore value, "How would your workout be different if you did test?". Joe says he knows he wouldn't crash as much, and his blood sugar would be more even. He'd have more energy. The coach uses the importance ruler. How important is it to test his blood glucose before his workouts? Joe replies it's an 8. The coach looks for more value - "what makes it and eight and not a five?" Joe says when he gets one low, he's apt to get another, and he doesn't like the yoyo effect. He says it's hard to get his glucose up without overshooting. He knows where he needs his glucose level to be when he begins his workout to avoid a 'low' and if he tests, he'll know whether he should eat a quick snack or sip some Gatorade during class.

Notice the coach doesn't need to understand anything about how Joe self manages his blood glucose. Joe is the expert! He knows exactly what to do. Helping him consider the value of what he wants to do will help him develop a plan to remember his meter and make the decision to test even when he doesn't feel like it.

Let's say Joe doesn't know much about his meter or how he can use information about his glucose levels to manage his diabetes better. He tells his coach his diabetes educator told him to test his glucose before and after his workouts, but he doesn't know how it will help him. In that case, the coach would explore what Joe wants to know and how he can get the information he needs.

Interrupting

Sometimes clients keep talking, and you don't want to be rude and interrupt! Because we want to listen and be respectful, interrupting is hard. It feels impolite, but it is sometimes necessary. We want to follow our clients but we need to manage the coaching process. I have never had a client get upset that I interrupted.

Occasionally a client will get really offtrack, sharing a story that has nothing to do with their health goals. To interrupt, you can say something like, "that sounds marvelous, and I'd love to hear more, but I want to make sure we have time to go over your health goals", you can soften it too by asking, "would that be ok?"

More often, clients are enthusiastic and get on a roll. What are the nuggets? What key things did the client tell you? Ask, "I just want to pause for a moment because you've said several things that pop out - that you want a better work-life balance, and while family time is important, you want to be able to have some time to yourself."

Another clue to interrupt is when a client is repeating information. You want to interrupt both to manage time and to highlight what the client is telling you. Ask, "can we pause right there because you said something really interesting," and then reflect, "you mentioned several times how little time you have to yourself," or "you've mentioned several times how much easier it would be if you had more help."

Interrupting is difficult but key to managing time, finding and keeping focus, and highlighting what is important to the client. Like everything in health coaching, it just takes practice.

Pause

We've been discussing talking and interrupting. Equally important is pausing. Pausing creates silence, and that can feel uncomfortable. In a conversation, when you have a pause, one party or the other will want to fill the silence and say something. In health coaching, pauses can be powerful. They hold space for the client to think. They can also prompt a client to say more. As the coach, you want to be mindful of pauses so you don't respond too quickly. Let a word or phrase sit a moment.

Practice pausing by using just reflections - "you've mentioned several times how much easier it would be if you had more help." Wait - see how the client responds.

Try counting in your head. It can feel like a long time but try counting to five - or ten - before you say anything. Try this in your everyday conversations. See what happens!

Good Reflections and Powerful Questions

Pauses can also help you compose better reflections and questions. I see many new coaches 'think out loud' as they respond to a client with a reflection or question. 'Thinking out loud,' the coach ends up repeating everything the client just said: "I hear you say you'd really like more time alone and that you have so much to do. You want more work-life balance, and that means getting more help from your family, but you aren't sure how to do that." Instead, you want to pick out the most important thing the client has told you. A more concise reflection that highlights what might be most important would be, "to get that balance, you're going to need help." Then wait, or ask, "What would balance look like?".

Powerful questions and reflections come from active listening. When you are genuinely listing to your client without jumping ahead with your own thoughts, you will hear what is most important to your client. You will hear how they interpret their circumstance, what they believe. When you hear what your client needs, you can ask questions and make reflections that are pertinent to your client's experience. This is also why it is better not to say "this is important to you," and instead say why it's important to your client. Instead of "it's important to have some time by yourself" say, "you need some time where you're not thinking about anyone else." Like many clients, this client expresses she feels guilty taking time for herself. Guilty is a big word - reflect it back. "Guilty" or "tell me about guilty" or "alone time without guilt." Listen for these meaning laden words - they are powerful words because they reflect what is impactful to your client.

Intonation

Listen to how you voice your reflections. Rising intonation - when your voice pitches up at the end of the sentence - will make your reflection sound like a question. You want to eat more *vegetables*? Instead you want to use falling intonation, keeping your pitch down makes it a statement. You want to eat more vegetables!

Education vs. Coaching

Presenting information and health coaching can go together, but they should be kept distinct and within the scope of practice. Health coaches are often asked to present information to clients as part of health initiatives or disease management programs where the employer has a specific protocol for you to follow. You may be directed to share information on the benefits of exercise, healthy eating, meditation, problem-solving, or tracking medication. The information can be valuable to clients. The key is presenting the information in a way that will not dictate the direction of the coaching portion of the session. If you can lead with the coaching and offer the information portion after the coaching, it will help keep the information you share from driving the coaching.

Often a wellness program or workshop will have educational pieces for each session. For example, a health coach is required to present ideas for making healthy choices when eating out. A client has had a heart attack and wants to learn how to cook heart-healthy meals at home. You can begin the session with what is most important to the client - cooking heart-healthy meals at home, and after the coaching portion is over, present the education portion of the session - making healthy choices when eating out. Frame it as distinct from the client's goal (of cooking at home): "So you have your plan for this week. Now, if it's ok, I have some information that's part of this wellness initiative about making healthy choices when eating out." Asking if the client wants the information before offering it keeps the client in the driver's seat. Then the coach can share the information the program requires.

Your employer may insist on a specific order for your presentation, but if you can coach first, you better ensure you are following the client's needs and keep the educational or information portion from driving the coaching session's direction.

Education can be a good marketing hook. Potential clients may not know what health coaching is but like the idea of learning about how to reduce stress or become change agents. The information you present needs to be something you are qualified to talk about, or you can partner with another professional. If it's a specific topic, like stress reduction, you will have a subject that will define the general coaching goal. People will come because they want to learn about how to reduce stress. You'll have the education part - how meditation can reduce stress with the individual or group participating in a guided meditation - and the coaching part - how can you begin meditating? In the next meeting, you start with a follow-up coaching portion, an educational piece, then end with coaching around the goals for the next week. I created a group coaching 'class' called Realizing Your Health Potential that I taught for a couple of years. Based on what we do in health coaching, it began with an introduction to the wheel of health, followed by segments on positive goal making, the mind-body connection, the stages of change, and the need for structure in SMART goals and action plans. Use what you know (and is within scope) to create your concept to combine education with coaching.

What Hat Are You Wearing?

When we follow our clients, listening for what they want to achieve for their health and how they might get there, we have to put aside our ideas about what they should do and where they should pay attention. This can be especially challenging when you are a health care practitioner.

Health coach training will help any health care practitioner be more effective. Practicing active listening, using motivational interviewing skills, partnering with patients, and meeting them where they are, makes healthcare more accessible and effective. Patients are heard, and their needs are better met. As a health coach, a health care professional wears two hats. One is the health expert hat (nurse, physician, dietitian, physical therapist, etc.) and the other is the health coach hat. When you wear the health care practitioner hat, you are the expert.

When you wear the health coach hat, the client is the expert. When you are a health care professional practicing as a health coach, clients will want to ask for your advice. Knowing when to keep on the coach hat and when to take it off is essential as "switching hats" can be both awkward and confusing and can derail the coaching session.

Let's consider a scenario where Edward sees his dietitian. Edward wants to avoid statins and goes to his dietitian to talk about diet changes to decrease his cholesterol. His dietitian, Susan, is a trained health coach. Susan begins the session in coaching mode, exploring Edward's health goals and what he thinks is important about making some diet changes. When she asks him, "what do you think would help you lower your 'bad' cholesterol?" Edward asks for advice. Susan thinks, ok, I'll be clear and ask permission to take off my coaching hat and put on my dietitian hat, and then I can offer some information. She says, "Edward, would it be ok if I take off my coach hat for a moment and put on my dietitian hat?". And Edward says yes! So Susan talks to him about what kinds of dietary changes might help him with his cholesterol goals. Now Susan is in her expert dietitian role, and all Edward has to do is ask her questions about what he should or should not eat.

And now we aren't coaching.

Once Susan puts on that dietitian hat, it's going to be very difficult for her to take it off. There is a power shift - Edward is no longer the expert - Susan is. She may be able to switch back, saying something like, "Given what I've just shared, what feels like some good next steps ?". But it can be very difficult to take off that expert hat.

My advice is to coach first. When Edward asks for advice, Susan can say something like, "I do have some ideas and resources that might help, and I'm happy to share them with you, but first, I'd like to hear what you think." Shift it back to the client. Let Edward share his ideas and what he feels like he needs. He likely knows already what he might change, but if that expert hat goes on too early, Susan will never know, and Edward's plan won't be his plan - it will be Susan's prescription, not Edward's ideas.

Health coaching is a new field, and many people still don't understand the professional health coach's role. We need to preserve health coaching's integrity as a distinct profession, especially as it is such a new field. So if Susan is presenting herself as a health coach, she really needs to keep the dietitian hat off. If she is a dietitian using health coaching skills to better help her patients that's great - but in that role she is a dietitian with health coach skills, not a health coach.

Non-health care professionals switch hats too! And the same advice holds true. Edward goes to another health coach, John, who drastically changed his health by eating vegan, and Edward wants to know how he did it!! If John leads with how eating vegan helped him lower cholesterol and glucose levels, it's now all about John - not Edward. John is the expert. Instead, John wants to keep off that expert hat (my experience as a vegan) and keep the health coach hat on tight. "Yes, you're right. I did make some changes that helped me with my health. It sounds like you want to make some real changes too - tell me how you see yourself getting there".

Going to a coach who has faced similar struggles can be inspiring but what worked for John may not work for Edward. Many of us come to health coaching because we have had powerful experiences in making changes to our health, or we are the person others come to for advice. Many of my students are surprised when they discover what health coaches do as change facilitators - they are also pleasantly surprised at how much more powerful health coaching is than giving advice. It is also vital to staying within your scope of practice.

The Value of Being "Coachy"

Your skills and knowledge as a health coach empower you to help others in reaching their goals. If you stay true to the spirit of health coaching, you can use this superpower in your other work as a health care practitioner, fitness trainer, community health worker, wellness coordinator, patient advocate, health educator, or anytime you are helping someone figure out how they can achieve their health goals.

Case Study: A Simple Solution

Matilda is meeting with her health coach in a follow-up session. She is fifty four and is on one medication to help manage her blood pressure - she would like to lose a few pounds and avoid any more medication. She has been building an exercise routine and eating more vegetarian meals, and she has succeeded with a prior goal of using a stand-up desk. She is a client that has some experience now working with her coach and finding what works for her.

Coach: Hi, Matilda! Good to see you again!

Matilda: Good to see you too!

Coach: Last time we met, you wanted to concentrate on your workouts. You've been going to your neighborhood gym to a small group workout class you like, and you've been trying to add some running. How did it go?!

Matilda: Good. My morning workouts have been going well - I go Tuesday and Thursday at 6:30. That's good. I got up to run on Monday both this week and last week, but I'm having a hard time getting up again on Wednesday to run. So I'll manage to run early once during the week, and on Saturday or Sunday, but it's hard to get up early more than two mornings.

Coach: You got four workouts done - two at the gym and two days running!

Matilda: Yes - and that's been for three weeks now!

Coach: That's awesome. Some difficulty with that one morning but the others working well. How does that feel?

Matilda: Great! I already feel stronger, and I like the people in the class.

Coach: Feeling great about those four workouts - what do you think about that third run?

Matilda: I think I'd like to hold off on that for now, but I would like to take the subway to work a couple of times a week - that would add two or three evening walks. My spouse can drop me off at the station in the morning, and then I can walk home.

Coach: Adding some extra walks instead of a third run. I don't want to forget your other goal - eating more vegetarian meals. How has that been going?

Matilda: Happy to say that is good too! And I've managed to avoid going out for lunch more than a couple of times.

Coach: That's great! Happy with your food choices, even eating out less! Getting your exercise done and adding the extra walks, what would be most helpful today? Would you like to look more at this, or something else?

Matilda: Actually, I'd like to look at something else. I want to find time to read more fiction.

Coach: Ok! Tell me more about that.

Matilda: I like to have a book goal, how many books I'll read in a year. And I like the quiet time, reading a good book, but in the evening, I want time to play piano, and now that I'm cooking some nights, that's less time to read. So I'm struggling with where to fit in some reading time.

Coach: Make sure you keep that reading time.

Matilda: Yes. I'm just not sure when.

Coach: Figuring out when you can sit down with a good book!

Matilda: Yes.

Coach: Tell me more about what it's like to be able to absorb yourself in a good story.

Matilda: It's nice quiet time, when I don't have to do anything else and to be able to just focus on reading. No other demands. It's relaxing.

Coach: Relaxing, with nothing else you have to do!

Matilda: Exactly. It's like a little refuge or mini-vacation that is there anytime I want it.

Coach: And having access to this mini-vacation helps balance your day.

Matilda: Yes - reading helps me de-stress. And it's fun!

Coach: So as you continue your exercise routine, and cook some more at home, and keep time to play piano, you need to have time to read too.

Matilda: Yes.

Coach: What can reading look like now?

Matilda: Well, I read the newspaper when I have coffee in the morning - I could read a book instead. But you know - I read a magazine at the office last week! I recently got rid of a second credenza in my office to make room for a table. It's a funny thing, but with the table I can sit down and eat lunch instead of eating at my computer. I didn't have a book, but I read a magazine. I should take a book to work - and I can read on the subway!

Coach: A few possibilities - reading a good book instead of the newspaper, reading at lunch, and when you take the subway. What do you think?

Matilda: They all sound good. I'll start packing my kindle to work, and I can read when I take the subway this week.

Coach: So reading at lunch and when you take the train, what about in the morning?

Matilda: Yes - I'll do that too. I hear enough news, and it's a nice way to start the day.

Coach: And you mentioned you have a yearly reading goal.

Matilda: I do, and I have a bunch of books ready on my kindle waiting for me.

Coach: On a scale from one to ten, with one being not at all confident, and ten being very confident, how confident are you about reading in the morning, with your coffee, when you take the subway, and at lunch?

Matilda: I'll say an eight. I would say a ten, but I may have a couple of days when I won't be at my office for lunch.

Coach: And what makes it an eight and not a five?

Matilda: I like it too much - as I said, it could be a ten!

Coach: Awesome! Anything else that might get in the way?

Matilda: I don't think so. I think I am set!

There are a few things to note in this case study. First, the coach checked in on what the client wanted the focus of the session to be - the session began by reviewing the client's experience with her exercise and healthy eating goals, then the coach checked in to make sure this is what the client wanted to continue to talk about. The focus shifted then to reading, and the coach took time to explore value - to see what reading does for the client? How is her life improved when she can read fiction? Then the coach checked in to see what ideas had surfaced, and the client identified three times she could read. When coaches take time to allow clients to explore and ponder what is important about the change they want to make, possibilities will surface. You can see here the opportunities were there - but only the client can identify what those opportunities are!

Stan and Edwina, Two Case Studies with Multiple Choice Questions

Stan

Stan has heart failure and has already met with his health coach once. Stan has been proactive about making some diet changes and is eager to work in more exercise. He has a wearable defibrillator (LifeVest) as his doctor assesses his condition. A wearable defibrillator protects people like Stan who are at risk of sudden cardiac death.

The case study is interspersed with multiple-choice answers. See how you do!

Coach: Hi, Stan! It's good to see you.

Stan: Hi, yes, same here.

Coach: How are you doing today?

Stan: Pretty good - I can't complain! The rain finally stopped.

Coach: Excellent! So things are drying out.

Stan: That's right. And with all that rain I couldn't get out as much as I wanted.

Coach: Yeah, so tell me more about last week - because one of your goals was to keep walking.

Stan: Yes, and I haven't been able to do much the last few days. Like yesterday, the rain tapered off in the morning, but it was so muggy. You know, I have to wear this LifeVest, so I try and get out early before it's too hot, so I missed a few days, but I did walk a mile this morning.

How should the coach respond?

A) What is a LifeVest?

B) How was it?

C) Oh, good - that's great!

D) It's important you walk every day.

The answer is B, "How was it?"

We don't really need to know what a LifeVest is (and you could look it up later). We also want to manage our time.

C is a fine affirmation, and you could go with that, while B holds the possibility of eliciting more while still acknowledging the walk. You could also combine them "Oh good - that's great! How was it?".

D is kind of bossy, and while it might reflect the client's goals, it sounds like the coach's opinion.

Coach: How was it?

Stan: Good! And this week looks a lot better.

Coach: You'll be able to get your walks in.

Stan: No doubt about it!

Coach: And when we met last week, you were keen to meet with your cardiologist to see what your ejection fraction is, and you are hoping to get some answers about your health and where you go next.

Stan: I see him Thursday. I'm kind of in limbo. I have a call scheduled with human resources to see what my options might be if I have to go on long-term disability.

What should the coach say next?

A) That's a really tough spot to be in.

B) You are thinking you will need long term disability.

C) With more information, you will know where you stand.

D) Tell me more about being in limbo.

Here C is the best response. It reflects his wish to gather more information from both his employer and cardiologist to gain a sense of what his next steps will be. It meets him where he is.

A is a reflection that highlights the negative - he's been pretty upbeat, so it feels gratuitous.

B reflects a what Stan is thinking, but does not move the coaching forward, especially as we are still exploring what Stan wants.   Also note that the coach would be jumping on the first train if they decided to ask Stan more about what he needs to know about long term disability!

D is an open question that also highlights the negative.

Coach: With more information, you will know where you stand.

Stan: Exactly. I'd like to know if I can go back to work, what's next - my e fraction, and when I can stop wearing this vest. And my daughters have been checking in on me - one lives nearby, and the other is up in Connecticut. They're helping me with some cooking ideas.

Coach: I remember last time you said you were eating more fish, that you've been trying some new healthy recipes.

Stan: Yes. And I like salmon. I like cooking too. It's just to get some of these ingredients, I have to go to two or three stores. It can be a lot of driving.

Which is best?

A) Having to drive around to get what you need.

B) Have you tried other types of fish?

C) Maybe you should try some easier recipes.

D) That is a lot of driving!

The answer is A. Again, A just meets Stan where he is. Driving to multiple stores may be bothersome, and it might be what he needs to do to get all of his groceries. We don't know. A more neutral reflection keeps the door open -Stan will likely tell us what he needs!

B is leading, and Stan hasn't said anything about other types of fish.

C is another suggestion and is also leading!

D is a reflection that acknowledges the downside of his shopping experience - it's better to go neutral and keep the door open. [22]

Coach: Having to drive around to get what you need.

Stan: Yeah, but it's ok. Once I get into a routine, it'll be more manageable.

Coach: Get into a groove.[23]

Stan: Yes. And sorting through what I have. I'm trying to have more fish, lean meats, more vegetables, and less salt. Some of the stuff in my pantry and freezer aren't what I want to eat anymore. And there's this no-salt seasoning I want to try.

What is the best response?

A) When can you start clearing out your pantry and freezer?

---

[22] You could follow with a double sided reflection, "On the one hand, you had to go to a few stores, on the other hand you were able to get what you needed", but it still sounds kind of flat.

[23] A nice positive refection, and it leaves the door open. Stan comes back with more - but if he just replied "yes" we could ask something like, "what would make it easier?"

B) There's a new normal to your way of eating and trying new things.

C) Have you tried eating vegan?

D) Yes, it's a good idea to avoid salt!

B is best, "there's a new normal to your way of eating and trying new things." It acknowledges the healthy change Stan is making, a new routine, a new normal in a positive way. [24]

A is going straight to action - too soon!

C is a suggestion and leading. It's also out of scope.

D highlights what the coach thinks is important. It's distracting from the rest of what the client said.

Coach: There's a new normal to your way of eating and trying new things.

Stan: Yes.

Coach: What's the seasoning?[25]

Stan: There's one by Norton and one from Penzance. I'll have to order them.

---

[24] Tone of voice makes a big difference - it's a good new normal as opposed to a bad new normal.

[25] Just a nice short engaging question is ok - we don't need the information but it is sowing interest and is unlikely to take us off track.

Coach: Very cool. So you are enjoying cooking and trying new things - it sounds like you've really embraced this new way of eating.

Stan: It's something I can do, and I do like to cook. I just usually don't have the time. Right now, I have lots of time!

Coach: Time to cook! And thinking about your long term goal to be healthy and as strong as you can be, except for the rain, you've been walking, finding and cooking healthy meals, and you have appointments with HR and your cardiologist so you can start to assess what your options will be—for the next week, continuing those?[26]

Stan: Yes - and I want to walk further. I do get tired, so I think I could add a shorter walk in the evening. And I want to finish some remodeling projects around the house.

Next?

A) Walking further would be good.

B) Maybe you should wait since you feel tired.

C) A nice evening walk, and what house project do you want to tackle first?

D) What are your remodeling projects?

C does the most here, "A nice evening walk, and what house project do you want to tackle first?", it acknowledges the walk and looks to pin down what house project Stan wants to do, moving the coaching along.

---

[26] We are shifting to action now.

A is the coach's opinion. A better reflection would be "a way to get some more walking without it being too taxing!"

B is a suggestion and seeks to limit the client's ambition.

D seeks more information without moving the coaching forward. C is better because it explores what action the client wants to make, what remodeling project he wants to work on the next week.

Coach: A nice evening walk, and what house project do you want to tackle first?

Stan: I put down a new floor a couple of years ago and never finished the shoe molding. That'll surprise my boyfriend too!

Coach: Excellent!

Stan: Yeah, I'm not always good at finishing the details! I won't tell Joe - it'll get a laugh!

Coach: Awesome! Any other home projects in mind?

Stan: Like I said, I need to get some of that food out of the house. I don't want to throw it away - maybe see what I can take to the food bank. Opened stuff I guess I'll need to throw away - I don't know if they take frozen dinners, stuff like that.

What should the coach say next?

A) Maybe your boyfriend can get rid of it for you?

B) Do you want to focus on getting rid of the food you don't want or finishing the shoe molding?

C) Taking the food to the food bank is a great idea!

D) Seeing what you can give away.

The best choice here is D. Seeing what you can give away. Again, it's a more neutral reflection, though, with the right inflection, it is affirmative.

A is really a suggestion.

B limits unnecessarily options, Stan might want to do both, and if you keep the options out there, Stan will tell you if he doesn't.

C is a fine affirmation, but the challenge is what he can take to the food bank.

Coach: Seeing what you can give away.

Stan: My daughter might take some of it too - I'll ask her first. That would be easy - she can just come and take what she wants, and I can see what's left to deal with.

Coach: Do you want to do that this week?[27]

Stan: Yes- I can call her this afternoon. She was going to come over tomorrow anyway. I'll make sure I have ice for the cooler too.

Coach: See how much she can take away for you!

Stan: Yes, she's a good daughter.

What's next?!

---

[27] A close question to check in on what action he will take.

A) That's terrific, and you said both daughters are giving you meal ideas. Cooking this week - do you know what you want to do?

B) That's so great your daughters are there to help you!

C) Who else might be able to help?

D) You want to have the cooler ready for her so she can take the frozen items.

A is best, "That's terrific, and you said both daughters are giving you meal ideas. Cooking this week - do you know what you want to do?." It acknowledges Stan's comment about his daughter, ties back to cooking, and then checks in to see if Stan knows what he wants to cook.

   B follows the client's statement about his daughter and would be a normal conversational reply, but in health coaching, we are being strategic, keeping in mind the coaching process and managing time, so A is better.

   C assumes he needs more help, and he hasn't indicated that he does.

   D is a reflection that does not move the coaching forward - we need to get to his SMART goals and action plan!

Coach: That's terrific, and you said both daughters are giving you meal ideas. Cooking this week - do you know what you want to do?

Stan: I have a shopping list - we'll go out to lunch tomorrow so I'll go shopping Wednesday. I know what I want to make.

Coach: Oh, good! So this week, more healthy cooking - getting the food you don't want in the house out - sounds like you are on a roll!

Stan: As I said, I have the time, and it just makes sense.

Coach: Absolutely. And you want to add a second short walk.[28]

Stan: Yes, I think that will be good.

Coach: So some good eating, good exercise. You have your appointments with the doctor and HR, so hopefully, you will have a better idea of what's next, and in the meantime finishing the shoe molding! Which it sounds like no one will expect![29]

Stan: Ha! Yes, that's right!

Coach: And you mentioned calling your daughter this afternoon about the food - and making extra ice for the cooler.[30]

Stan: Yes. And I'm going to order those spices.

Coach: Awesome! Do you need any reminders? For the evening walk - or materials for the floor?[31]

Stan: No - I have what I need. Hopefully, next week I won't have the LifeVest.

Coach: Fingers crossed! I look forward to seeing you next week!

---

[28] Touching back on adding exercise.

[29] Here is a summary of most of his goals.

[30] More action.

[31] Checking in on the reminder. We could do a summary more precisely defining his SMART goals but we have just touched on everything and his plan of action is clear. If there was any doubt expressed, or obstacles cited, we would take time to explore what else would help him succeed.

Edwina

Here is another case study with multiple choice answers! Edwina is seeing a health coach because she plans to have bariatric surgery. The hospital where she is being treated requires all bariatric patients to complete a series of sessions with a health coach before having surgery.

Coach: Hi, Edwina! Welcome! I'm glad you were able to come in today.

Edwina: Hi, thank you. I kind of have to, but this is fine.

Coach: Thank you for coming. My job here as a health coach is to support you as you get ready for your surgery. They have found here at the bariatric center that health coaching helps patients prepare for surgery and the changes that follow surgery. It's really about what will best support you as you go through this process. How does that sound?[32]

Edwina: That sounds good.

Coach: You've decided to take this next step - and have the surgery - how does it feel?

Edwina: Good. I just really want it to be done, but I know I have to do this and I'm supposed to lose thirty pounds before they will schedule it. So there's that.

---

[32] Here the coach is setting expectations and developing rapport - the client seems a bit uncertain, which is natural when it's not necessarily her choice to see the coach.

What should the coach say next? What is the best response?

A) Maybe you can lose enough weight you won't need the surgery.

B) Yes, it's imperative you lose that 30 pounds first.

C) Yes - so what can you do to lose that 30 pounds?

D) So there are some things you need to do before surgery.

The best response is D, "so there are some things you need to do before surgery."

A is leading, that could happen, but that is not why the client is here. This is an easy way to lose the client - instead, reflect to show you are listening - this will build trust. With "Maybe you can lose enough weight you won't need the surgery", Edwina might respond: "I've been on so many diets - all I do is gain more weight back", or "I didn't think that was why I am here" or "Yes I suppose that could happen" or "That would be nice." By inserting an opinion rather than following the client, the coach erodes trust and gives up an opportunity to build confidence and explore what is important to the client!

B sounds a little mean, doesn't it? It's because the coach is picking the agenda - rather than partnering with the client and listening, and the coach is choosing a pretty forceful word, IMPERATIVE!

C is a very common mistake new coaches make - it goes straight to action before taking time to explore value. We need to set the groundwork first - what is important to Edwina about having bariatric surgery? Going directly to acton also means we aren't taking time to see what else Edwina might want to focus on - we are setting the focus with the very first thing she says. We are 'jumping on the first train'. We want to take time - see what other trains might come by! All kinds of things might come up.

D is the best response. It's a simple reflection. It shows the coach is listening and follows the client's lead.

Let's continue -

Coach: So, there are some things you need to do before surgery.

Edwina: Yes. And I get it - I know that some people lose the weight just to end up putting it back on, or they eat poorly, and I need to lose some more weight so the surgery is safer.

What should the coach say next?

A) You know some of the possible dangers, and you want to do well in surgery, and you want to be smart about how you eat after surgery!

B) Yes, it can be easy to gain the weight back after surgery.

C) So especially important to understand what you need to do.

D) So, what do you need to make sure you eat well and keep off the weight after surgery?

The answer is A, "you know some of the possible dangers and want to do well in surgery, and you want to be smart about how you eat after surgery!" There is a lot here! We can see that Edwina has, not surprisingly, thought a lot about this and has some ideas about possible problems. There is value here too. She wants to do well in surgery; she wants to be smart about how she eats. Edwina is planning ahead, so she is prepared for what awaits her.

B is a reflection that focuses on her fear - it's not likely to move the coaching forward.

D goes straight to action! We are jumping on the first (or second) train!

C is okay, but A is better.

Coach: You know some of the possible dangers and want to do well in surgery, and you want to be smart about how you eat after surgery!

Edwina: Yes! I certainly don't want to go through all of this just to end up back at square one.

Coach: You want this to be a success story!

Edwina: Absolutely! I can do this! I've already lost ten pounds!

Coach: Fantastic!

Edwina: Thank you.

Coach: What helped you lose this first ten pounds?[33]

Edwina: I did the Daniel Fast at church - it's three weeks long and eating a lot of fruit and vegetables, fish, lots of healthy foods. I'm going to keep doing that to help me lose the other twenty pounds.

---

[33] Let's note there have been two reflections and an affirmation before the coach asks another question (what helped you lose this first ten pounds?). Remember, we want to use more reflections than questions. Also, by asking the client what worked, we bring attention to the client's strengths and success.

Which response is best?

A) What is the Daniel Fast?

B) Are you eating meat?

C) Perhaps you should see a dietitian first.

D) You've found something that really works for you.

This time it's D, "you've found something that really works for you".

In A, the coach is mining for information. (New coaches often do this when they don't know what to do). The client knows what the Daniel Fast[34] is - she's just told you. There are also no nutrition alarm bells here. Asking her to tell you more is just asking the client to tell you what she already knows - i.e., the client's job is not to educate you!

---

[34] I've seen many clients do the Daniel Fast. The Daniel Fast is inspired by the Bible's first book of David. Trepanowski and Bloomer studied the effects of the Daniel Fast. They write, "the Biblical-based Daniel Fast prohibits the consumption of animal products, refined carbohydrates, food additives, preservatives, sweeteners, flavorings, caffeine, and alcohol. It is most commonly partaken for 21 days, although fasts of 10 and 40 days have been observed. Our initial investigation of the Daniel Fast noted favorable effects on several health-related outcomes, including: blood pressure, blood lipids, insulin sensitivity, and biomarkers of oxidative stress." I have seen variations in what is or is not included, and clients do not always follow a strictly vegan interpretation - which is fine! We are not looking for clients to adhere to a certain diet - but to eat a healthy diet as defined by MyPlate.gov and the Academy of Nutrition and Dietetics (formerly the American Dietetic Association).

119

B is gratuitous and possibly leading - it sounds like the coach is fishing.

I question the reasoning for C - nothing the client has said raises any alarm. If the coach feels uncomfortable, they can check-in to see if the plan meets the recommendations on My Plate. Suggesting so early that the client might want to see a dietitian can undermine the client-coach relationship. The coach is also questioning the client's judgment without cause.

D is the best response - it's a reflection that meets the client where she is and affirms her success.

Coach: You've found something that really works for you.[35]

Edwina: Yes, I was surprised - it's pretty easy, and I got a lot of ideas about what to eat. As part of the fast, we get recipes and make some potluck dinners.

Coach: Short term, you know you need to lose twenty more pounds - already having lost ten with the help of the Daniel Fast. What other short - or long - term goals do you have?

Edwina: Well, long term, I want to lose a hundred and twenty pounds! But short term, I know I need to start exercising, but I don't know......I've never been an exerciser.

---

[35] You could ask more about what other ideas or tools she has learned with the Daniel Fast - sometimes that jogs a client's memory and inspires more action - but we also have to manage our time. This is an area where the client seems pretty confident, so instead we will check in on what else she wants to do.

A) You've never seen yourself as an exerciser, and this is a great time to start!

B) Exercising is scary.

C) Exercising is something you don't really feel confident about, but you think it would be beneficial.

D) What kind of physical activity do you enjoy?

What is the best response?

C is best, "exercising is something you don't really feel confident about, but you think it would be beneficial."

A is a reflection that likely misses the mark. It is also directive - i.e., the coach thinks this is a great time to start!. Listen for where the client is in the stages of change - she is in contemplation, perhaps even tenuously in contemplation - if you push her to action she is more likely to fail.

B is another reflection, but this one projects a negative that will not lead the coaching forward. The client didn't say exercise is scary (but a coach might project that). She said she doesn't identify as an exerciser.

D goes right to action, ignoring the client's hesitation and uncertainty. This is heavy-handed and ignores where the client is.

C, "Exercising is something you don't really feel confident about but thinking that perhaps it's something that would be beneficial" is the best response. It is a double-sided reflection, first acknowledging the negative or uncertainty and then stating the upside but in a relatively neutral way- not trying to push the client to action but inviting her to share why she thinks exercising might be helpful. We are following the client's lead but not pushing her.

Coach: Exercising is something you don't really feel confident about but thinking that perhaps it's something that would be beneficial.

Edwina: Yes.

Coach: What else is important to you - to realize that success of 120 pounds?![36]

Edwina: Like I said, keeping it off. I should lose it pretty quickly after the surgery, and other patients have lots of tips . I guess I'm kind of worried about how I'll eat after the surgery. You can only have a little food at a time, and you have to be careful about how much water you drink too. Everybody knows I'm doing the surgery, so I'm not concerned about going out or anything, but yeah, I guess the nitty-gritty about what I can eat.

What's next?

A) Would it help if I went over this handout I have on your first year after bariatric surgery?

B) What if you made a list of your questions to take to your next appointment at the center?

C) You think it would help you to have a clear picture of what eating and drinking will look like after surgery.

---

[36] We could decide to talk more about exercise here but the coach is checking in to see if there are other more pressing goals or areas where the client feels more confident. Remember - we want to avoid jumping on the first train! We can come back to exercise later as we define the focus.

D) You're comfortable going out even though you can't eat like everybody else.

C is best, "You think it would help you to have a clear picture of what eating and drinking will look like after surgery".

A jumps right to education/information. It could also be out of scope though someone working with a bariatric/weight loss program might be trained to share such information, but the coach is shifting quickly to an expert role. Instead let's see first what the client needs.

B is suggestive and leading - you might have tools for the client to consider, but this is not the time to share.

D is kind of a backhanded affirmation and misses what to highlight in a reflection. C is the best response. It is a reflection that summarizes what the client has said.

Coach: You think it would help you to have a clear picture of what eating and drinking will look like after surgery.

Edwina: Yes - I want to know exactly how much I should eat, and if there is anything I shouldn't eat. And the whole thing about drinking and eating at the same time.

Coach: Because right now some things are a bit fuzzy, and if you had more information, you'd know what it is you need to do.

Edwina: Right - there are still some pieces I'm not sure about.

Coach: You know you want to have more information about what you can expect after surgery.

Edwina: Yes.

Coach: If it's okay, let me see if I can summarize what we've talked about so far. One hundred twenty pounds is your ultimate target, and doing the Daniel Fast at church has helped you lose ten pounds and continuing it will help you lose another twenty. It also sounds like it has given you a lot of good ideas about new things to try. You mentioned you should maybe do some exercise and that you definitely want to more the details about eating after surgery. Is that right?[37]

Edwina: Yes, exactly!

What's the best response?

---

[37] We have three reflections followed by a summary (which is also a type of reflection). More reflections are always better - it's hard to go astray when you reflect! Reflections should not simply say what the client told you but help move the coaching along. The coach could say "you're not sure about how food and drink go together," which just highlights the negative and does not help move the coaching forward - and a chain of negative reflections can easily shift the coaching into a downward spiral! You also don't want to insert positive reflections that aren't true to what the client has told you. Instead, acknowledge the problem "Because right now there are some things that are a bit fuzzy', and then reflect the positive, "and if you had more information you'd know what it is you need to do". The summary let's us figure out what the focus should be - is it the Daniel Fast? Exercise? Or getting information about what to expect after surgery? All three? Or something else? Edwina confirms the summary - let's further define the focus, see where we need to explore value more (ie, esp in those areas where there is uncertainty (contemplation) before we move to action. What we know so far is Edwina seems quite confident about the Daniel Fast, contemplative and uncertain about exercise and feeling a need for more information, but we don't know yet if that information is easy or hard for her to find.

124

A) So we are going to design an action plan for you for the next two weeks - which of these goals do you want to focus on?

B) And finding a way to get in some exercise will help you lose the twenty pounds even faster!

C) Anything else that you think would help?

D) So, definitely continuing the Daniel Fast - what will that look like these next two weeks?

The answer is C, "Anything else that you think would help?"

A is limiting and feels pushy - and it's assuming the client is ready to act with a plan. Better would be to explore more - is there something else out there - something else Edwina is thinking about? Coaching is built on trust. When clients realize you are truly listening to what they want, and that you are not judging them for what they are struggling to do, they feel more confident about sharing goals, aspirations, fears, and difficult emotions. If you were really pressed for time, you could say something like, "We have just a bit of time left, that would help you most?" (the Daniel Fast, looking at exercise or finding the information you want post surgery?).

B is leading!

D could be fine, especially if time is short, and as long as the coach checks back on the other two items: exercise and post-surgery information.

C is best because it takes time to check-in and makes sure these are the topics the client wants to address.

Coach: Anything else that you think would help?

125

Edwina: No, that's it - what happens after surgery - and I'm supposed to be doing a workout plan. They gave us information at the bariatric center and a three-month membership to the gym.

What should the coach say next?

A) Right, and you're not sure about that.

B) The doctor really wants you to go to the gym.

C) What do you see yourself doing at the gym?

D) How would things be different if you were able to work out at the gym?

It's A, "right, and you're not sure about that". A acknowledges that uncertainty the client expressed earlier.

D is a good value question, but notice it goes right to 'working out at the gym' - if you ask a value question about a topic where it appears the client is in contemplation you want to ask it in a way that opens opportunities. Instead of asking about the gym ask something like "how would having more physical activity help?", or even "what would be different if you were able to exercise?". I like to avoid jargon or loaded terms when possible - a 'gym' can bring up all kinds of expectations as can the idea of a 'workout'.

C is going right to action - too soon!

B overreaches - the doctor probably does want Edwina to go to the gym, but that is unlikely an effective source of motivation! What does Edwina want?!

A shows the coach is listening and picks up on the client's uncertainty. This can move the coaching into exploring what exercise or physical activity might mean for the client, whether the client sees value in exercise, and if she might be ready to act in some form (which may or may not include the gym or a prescribed workout).

Coach: Right, and you're not sure about that.

Edwina: Yes. I don't know why it seems so hard.[38]

Coach: What would be different if you could do it? If you had that regular exercise routine?

Edwina: I'd probably lose more weight. I know it's supposed to make you feel better and more muscle burns more calories. I'd like to be more fit. Be able to do more. But, yeah, I don't know.

Coach: Tell me more about being able to do more.

Edwina: Do things with ease - everything would just be easier.

Coach: Life would be easier.

Edwina: Yes. Life would be easier. That's why I want the surgery to help me lose all this extra weight.

What should the coach say next?

A) So exercise really is important to you.

---

[38] It's hard because she is not ready to act - or the action she envisions isn't something she wants or feels able to do. This tells you she is in contemplation.

B) So if you could exercise - use that free membership - you'd not only lose weight, but all kinds of things would be easier!

C) You know what you want - and you've made real steps already to get to your goal of losing a hundred and twenty pounds - which will make all kinds of things easier. Tell me more about what this will look like - when you've met this big goal?

D) You've had success with the Daniel Fast - what has that taught you about what would make it easier to go to the gym? To use that free membership?!

C is best, "You know what you want - and you've made real steps already to get to your goal of losing a hundred and twenty pounds - which will make all kinds of things easier. Tell me more about what this will look like - when you've met this big goal?"

A is a reflection that misses the mark - is exercise really important to Edwina? She would like the effects of exercise, but this implies she values exercise in her life. Better would be something like, "You can see there would be some real benefits to exercise." It's also good to avoid saying "(x) is important to you". Instead, substitute "important" for what you've heard, like "having more exercise would allow you to move with ease" or "You think exercise could help you both lose weight and feel better". Hearing what is important is more powerful.

B is pushing that free membership! It's tone-deaf - again, let's keep it open - Edwina may or may not want to go to the gym. D begins well - it's a question seeking to tap into the client's strengths - what has helped her be successful? But here again, the question narrows the focus to the gym.

C affirms the client's success, reflects value, and follows with a vision question that can elicit more value.

Coach: You know what you want - and you've made real steps already to get to your goal of losing a hundred and twenty pounds - which will make all kinds of things easier. Can you tell me more about what this will look like - when you've met this big goal?

Edwina: Sure - I mean, I will be able to do more and feel more confident, more energized. I want to be healthy.

Coach: More confident, more energy, good health! What else?[39]

Edwina: I'll feel better about myself. Proud!

Coach: Proud. (pause)

Edwina: Yes! I'll be proud of myself - I am proud of what I've done already!

Coach: Awesome!

Edwina: Yes - proud!

Which response is next?

A) Thinking about what you have accomplished already, and thinking specifically about what steps you want to take these next two weeks, what will you do in terms of exercise?

---

[39] The coach has followed with a pretty basic reflection - that works well here. It is often powerful for clients to hear back big emotive value statements or words: confidence, energy, good health! Of course, what words or phrases are powerful will be different for each client. When you listen you will hear what is meaningful to your client, allowing you to respond with powerful questions and reflections.

B) Thinking about what you have accomplished already and thinking specifically about what steps you want to take these next two weeks, You want to do the Daniel Fast, and you want to exercise.

C) Thinking about what you have accomplished already and thinking specifically about what steps you want to take these next two weeks, what do you want to accomplish? You mentioned continuing the Daniel Fast.

D) What else will make you proud?!

C is the answer,   "Thinking about what you have accomplished already and thinking specifically about what steps you want to take these next two weeks, what do you want to accomplish? You mentioned continuing the Daniel Fast."

A goes right back to exercise! We've just heard some great value/ change talk - we risk diminishing that by going back to a particular action where we already know there is uncertainty.

B includes the Daniel Fast but also narrows the focus to exercise.

D feels more like misguided fishing rather than following the client.

C is now moving to action - we have laid the groundwork, let's see what the client is ready to do.

Coach: Thinking about what you have accomplished already and thinking specifically about what steps you want to take these next two weeks, what do you want to accomplish? One thing was continuing the Daniel Fast.[40]

Edwina: Yes.

Coach: That was something you were doing through your church, visualizing continuing that now, especially into the next two weeks, is there anything that might get in the way?

Edwina: I'm going away for the weekend - but there are enough options that I can pretty much eat anywhere, and I'll be taking food with me too. And there is a group of us who want to keep it up so we can, you know, support each other.

What's next?

A) Excellent - you already have a plan!

B) So you've already thought about some next steps.

C) That's wonderful. It's so important to have the support of your friends.

D) Would you like me to share a handout I have with tips for making healthy choices when eating at a restaurant?

Here, B is best, "So you've already thought about some next steps."

D is leading. Does she need advice for ordering in restaurants? That said, a coach working in a weight loss program might have relevant

---

[40]Continuing the Daniel Fast was an action the client expressed early, and with confidence - the coach is checking in to see if there are any possible obstacles.

131

information to share and can be within scope if it is not dietary advice. In that case asking the client permission to share is appropriate but take care not to derail the coaching with education. I suggest asking to share information at the end of the session so it does not drive the session.

C is not following the client, sure it is important to have supportive friends, but this may or may not resonate with the client.

A is a bit too early - does she have a plan?

B is acknowledging what the client has done and leaves space for the client to offer more.

Coach: So you've already thought about some next steps.

Edwina: Yes, absolutely.

Coach: On a scale from one to ten, one being not confident at all and ten being very confident - how confident are you that you can continue the Daniel Fast these next two weeks?

Edwina: Oh, that's a nine - I'd say ten, but I want to leave a little wiggle room!

Coach: Awesome - and what makes it a nine and not a six?[41]

Edwina: I'm used to it now, and I know what I need to do.

---

[41] Asking the client what makes it a higher number and not a lower number encourages her to reflect on her strengths and on what she has already achieved. This would be true even if her number was lower (what makes it a six and not a two?) This is an easy way to elicit more value/change talk.

Next?

A) And you mentioned getting information for after surgery - is that something you want to look into now?

B) So let's go over what you need to do.

C) Do you mind if we go over what you need to do to stay on the Daniel Fast?

D) Excellent! Sounds like a great plan!

The coach has to make a judgement call - we are nearing the end of the session, what do have left to do?

B and C are unlikely to elicit anything new and do not move the coaching along.

D skips defining the SMART goal and action plan and neglects checking in on the client's other goals: information about what she should do after surgery and exercise.

A is best. The client is very confident about her eating plan. She has already had success and she has a strategy for her trip. It's time to move on.

Coach: And you mentioned getting information for after surgery - Is that something you want to look into now?

Edwina: Yes, and I can do that at my next appointment, next month.

Coach: Perfect - do you need anything to help you remember what you want to ask?

Edwina: I'll make a note on my calendar reminder. You know, I can email the PA too. Let her know I have some questions. I've heard about it in the support group meetings, but I want to know exactly what I should expect.

Coach: Right - and this will give you the opportunity to talk one on one with the PA about it.

Edwina: Exactly.

Coach: And you mentioned exercise. It sounds like you're not quite sure what exercise you would do, but thinking some exercise would be beneficial.[42]

Edwina: Yes, but you know what, I need to do that. It'll help me lose weight and get to my goal more quickly, but I don't know about going to the gym. They mentioned some classes.

What should the coach say next?

A) Okay - you've heard about some classes. What are your thoughts about that?

B) You're thinking working out is important because it will help you lose the weight more quickly.

C) You've heard about classes, what feels like a do-able way to start to get in some exercise?

D) What would help you feel better about going to the gym?

---

[42] Here the coach is touching back on exercise by using a double sided reflection - notice we finish with the positive - this encourages change talk.

This time C is best, "you've heard about classes, what feels like a do-able way to start to get in some exercise?"

A is jumping on the exercise class train - this may or may not be something the client wants to do, and she may feel pushed to pick a class. We want to client to lead us to the solution.

B is an accurate reflection and revisits value but isn't likely to lead to any insight.

D is pushy - does she need to go to the gym?

C gives a nod to the new information about classes and asks the client what she could do - but keeps it open. Edwina might go to class or have a totally different idea about what she wants to do.

Coach: You've heard about classes, what feels like a do-able way to start to get in some exercise?

Edwina: Not the gym. I just don't know who will be there or what I will be able to do.

Coach: Some exercise, physical activity, not at the gym.

Edwina: Yes.

Coach: What would that be?[43]

Edwina: Oh, I could walk more. When I lived in New York City, I walked everywhere! But living here, you have to drive - that's when I started gaining weight!

---

[43] The coach can see that the gym is pretty iffy - this opens it up - what ideas does the client have?!

Which is best?

A) I hear that all the time! Do you have someplace you could walk?

B) Walking is something you used to enjoy.

C) You used to be more active, and now you aren't.

D) One of the reasons you gained weight was not being able to walk.

The answer is B, "Walking is something you used to enjoy."

A is going straight to action (and with a close-ended question) - we don't know how confident she is about walking.

C and D are negative and are likely to elicit sustain talk - i.e. what she is not doing.

B is picking up on the client's enthusiasm - here the coach is making a pretty easy guess that the client used to enjoy walking in NYC.

Coach: Walking is something you used to enjoy.

Edwina: I did, and you know I can walk - I can walk after work. That'd be nice.

Coach: Walking after work! Is that something you'd like to have as a goal for these next two weeks?[44]

Edwina: Yes, and I can at least do a walk around the block.

Coach: A nice walk around the block after work.

Edwina: Yes.

Coach: Workdays? Weekends? What are you thinking?

Edwina: I'll say every day - then see where that takes me.

Coach: Awesome! We are about out of time but let me see if I can summarize - these next two weeks, you will enjoy a walk every day. You will continue the Daniel Fast and you have some concrete ideas about what will make that easier when you are away at the beach. You already have an appointment with the PA at the bariatric center, and you can use that opportunity to get the information you need for after surgery - and you mentioned putting a reminder on your calendar and emailing the PA.

Edwina: That's right.

Coach: When would you want to email?

Edwina: I'll call them today - they might have something they can send me too.

Coach: Great! So checking with them today.

Edwina: Yes - I'll do that this afternoon

---

[44] The coach uses a quick close-ended question checking in to see if this is something she wants to do this week - alternatively, the coach could ask, "What does walking after work look like ?"

Coach: And walking around the block every day, anything that might get in the way? Or do you need a reminder?

Edwina: Just the weather, but it is supposed to be sunny. I think I'll remember, but I'll use my phone to remind me.

Coach: Excellent! Continuing the Daniel Fast, emailing the PA and walking! I look forward to seeing you next time and hearing more!

Appendix

Wheel of Health Worksheet

The Wheel of Health is a useful tool illustrating a whole person approach to health, and how different areas of our life inter-relate to create good health. Identifying your health values and goals and how they overlap can help you create an effective plan to achieve your health goals.

The Wheel of Health is made of eight spokes: physical activity, rest and relaxation, food and nutrition, finance, spirituality, occupation/ fulfilling work, relationships, and physical environment. Use this worksheet to describe your health vision. What are your health goals? Where are you now, and where would you like to be?

When you have completed the worksheet list the areas where you would like to make some changes. Where would you like to focus first?

Physical activity

Physical activity and how we move include exercise, daily movement, stretching, strength building, endurance, balance, and mobility. What is important to you about physical activity - what would you like to achieve in six months? Where would you like to be in a year?

Rest and relaxation

Rest and relaxation include getting good sleep, having downtime, or doing something just because it is relaxing and fun. It might mean getting away and going on vacation or time to enjoy a hobby. What is important to you about rest and relaxation? Where would you like to achieve in six months? Where would you like to be in a year?

Food and nutrition

Healthy eating, access to fresh foods, having the cooking skills to make meals at home. Meeting nutritional needs but also enjoying food. How do you feel about how you eat? Where would you like to be in six months? Where would you like to be in a year?

Finance

Financial security, financial planning. Having the money you need for shelter, food, transportation, education, savings, relaxation and travel. What are you financial goals? Where would you like to be in six months or a year?

Spirituality

Spiritual fulfillment, faith, connectedness to something other or greater than one's self. What are your thoughts about where you are spiritually? Where would you like to be spiritually in six months? Where would you like to be in a year?

Occupation/Fulfilling Work

Occupation/fulfilling work Work that provides intellectual stimulation and satisfaction, whether paid or volunteer work, a career pursuit, or a hobby. Thinking about fulfilling work, how do you feel about where you are now? Where would you like to be in six months? Where would you like to be in a year?

Relationships

Family, friends, community, relating to others, and relationships that are supportive and nurturing. Relationships can be fluid and shift over time. How do you feel about the relationships you have now? Where would you like to be in six months? Where would you like to be in a year?

Physical environment

A safe and comfortable home, neighborhood and surrounding community, access to transportation and other needs, as well as nature. What is important to you about your physical environment? What would you like to see in six months? Where would you like to be in a year?

Stress Reduction and Mindful Awareness

Mindful awareness: paying attention to the present moment, on purpose and without judgment. And we all know what stress is! Stress, particularly bad stress, can raise blood pressure, blood sugars, and make us more prone to illness. Mindful awareness allows us to be more present and focused and helps shut off stressful (and often critical) chatter in our heads.

Have you ever gotten caught up in a thought, finding you missed your exit on the highway? Or looked down at your plate and wondered where all the food went? We all tune out or got caught up in distraction. Being mindful breaks you out of distraction as you give attention to the present moment. Being mindful benefits our health, our relationships and helps us listen to ourselves and others.

Try being more mindful in your daily life. Spend a meal eating mindfully, noticing your food's color and smell, and how the flavor explodes in your mouth. Outside, notice how the sun feels on your skin, listen to the sounds around you. Pay attention to everyday tasks like washing dishes or taking a shower. Likewise, listen to your body - are your shoulders tense? Can you relax them?

You can be more mindful anywhere, anytime! Here are mindfulness exercises to try.

Paced Breathing

Our breathing becomes more rapid and shallow when we are stressed. By intentionally slowing your breath, you cue your body to relax. Meditation is often centered on the breath as it helps us relax and focus on the moment. For this paced breathing exercise, remember 4/7/8. Breath in through the nose for a count of four, hold the breath for a count of seven, and exhale through the mouth for a count of eight. If that feels too long, try holding your breath twice as long as you inhale and exhale about the same about of time as held

148

your breath. Try three of these deep breaths, you can do this exercise anytime, anywhere!

Mental Vacation

Here you imagine a pleasant destination. It can be someplace real, like a favorite vacation spot, or someplace you imagine you'd like to go.

Comfortably seated or lying down, close your eyes or softly gaze down, and think of a place - real or imagined - that you would like to visit during your mental vacation. A beach, sitting around a campfire, park, a cozy den — anyplace you'd like to go. Consider your surroundings, look around. Is there a breeze at your vacation spot? Warm sun? What sounds are there? Is there laughter, a crackling fireplace, or the sound of ocean surf? What's beneath your feet? Fall leaves or sand? Plush carpet or warm stone? Spend some time there, enjoying this favorite spot. Then, when you are ready, open your eyes and remember that this vacation spot is always available for you to visit!

Body Scan

Here your focus is on the body, moving your attention from your feet to your head. If your attention wanders, gently bring the focus back to the body. If you notice pain or discomfort, try to just notice. You aren't going to change what is there though easing tension by mindfully relaxing muscles can tension and related discomfort. If you lay down for this exercise, you may be more comfortable with a pillow beneath your knees.

Sit or lay down in a comfortable place and close or gently lower your eyes. Notice how your body is resting and supported, and take a few deeps breaths. Next, bring your attention to the body, focus on your feet. What do you notice? What sensations do you feel? If there is pain or discomfort, simply notice, observing what is. Now bring your attention to your legs. What do you notice? Imagine any tension dissolving and floating away, leaving the body. Now continue to your hips, back, and abdomen, arms, hands, shoulders, and neck, taking time to bring attention to each and relaxing any tension or tightness. Last, bring your attention to your head, noticing any sensations, relaxing your jaw, cheeks, and brow. Now, as you bring your body scan to a close, spend a few moments feeling your body as a whole, gently open your eyes or raise your gaze, and if you like, enjoying a nice stretch!

Meditation

A more 'formal' practice of meditation can bring you even more benefits. Meditation can boost your immune system, lower blood pressure, and reduce stress.

Guided meditations lend structure and offer variety to your meditation practice and are especially helpful for new meditators. There are many resources for recorded, guided meditations. Subscription plans like Headspace and Ten Percent Happier offer a variety of guided meditations and can be a good way to introduce yourself or clients to meditation. Free guided meditations are online - Jon Kabat-Zinn is on YouTube. Here are some to check out or share:

University of California Los Angeles Health: https://www.uclahealth.org/marc/mindful-meditations

University of California San Diego Medical School's Center for Mindfulness: https://medschool.ucsd.edu/som/fmph/research/mindfulness/pages/default.aspx

The Center for Contemplative Mind in Society: http://www.contemplativemind.org/practices/recordings

Tara Brach, a meditation teacher and psychotherapist in Washington D.C.: https://www.tarabrach.com/guided-meditations/

Mindful magazine: https://www.mindful.org/category/meditation/guided-meditation/

New York Times: https://www.nytimes.com/guides/well/how-to-meditate

A great list or resources and link from Stanford Medicine: https://wellmd.stanford.edu/content/dam/sm/wellmd/documents/Mindfulness-resources-10-2015.pdf

Another great resource is the eight-week Mindfulness-Based Stress Reduction (MBSR) program developed by Jon Kabat-Zinn. Mindfulness-Based Stress Reduction workshops should be lead by a qualified teacher. These can be in person or online, and there is usually a fee.

There is a free online MBSR class offered by Dave Potter at Palouse Mindfulness: https://palousemindfulness.com

An excellent MBSR workbook is A Mindfulness-Based Stress Reduction Workbook by Bob Stahl and Elisha Goldstein et al.

More Resources

Changing For Good by James Prochaska, John Norcross and Carlo DiClemente

Changing to Thrive: Using the Stages of Change to Overcome the Top Threats to Your Health and Happiness by James Prochaska & Janice Prochaska.

Full Catastrophe Living (Revised Edition): Using the Wisdom of Your Body and Mind to Face Stress, Pain, and Illness by Jon Kabat-Zinn

Living a Healthy Life with Chronic Conditions: Self-Management of Heart Disease, Arthritis, Diabetes, Depression, Asthma, Bronchitis, Emphysema and Other Physical and Mental Health Conditions, by Kate Lorig et al (also available on CD)

The Happiness Advantage: The Seven Principles of Positive Psychology that Fuel Success and performance at Work by Shawn Achor

Authentic Happiness: Using the New Positive Psychology to Realize Your Potential for Lasting Fulfillment by Martin E.P. Seligman

10% Happier: How I Tamed the Voice in My Head, Reduced Stress Without Losing My Edge, and Found Self-Help That Actually Works--A True Story, by Dan Harris

References

Al Muammar A.M, Ahmad Z, Aldamash AM. (2018) Paradigm Shift in Healthcare Through Technology and Patient-Centeredness. International Archives of Public Health and Community Medicine 2:015.

Advisory Board. (2019) 'There's Something Terribly Wrong', Why More Americans are Dying in Middle Age. Daily Briefing, December 2, 2019.

Boccia M, Piccardi L, Guariglia P. (2015) The Meditative Mind: A Comprehensive Meta-Analysis of MRI Studies. BioMed Research International, 2015;2015.

Center for Disease Control and Prevention. (1999) Achievements in Public Health, 1900-1999: Control of Infectious Diseases. Morbidity and Mortality Weekly, 1999/48(29);621-629.

Fredrickson, Barbara. (2010) Positivity: Top-Notch Research Reveals the 3 to 1 Ratio That Will Change Your Life. Crown Publishing.

Marsh, Jason. (2011) A Little Meditataion Goes a Long Way. Greater Good Magazine, Science-Based Insights for a Meaningful Life, February 2, 2011.

McGonigal, Kelly. (2011) The Willpower Instinct: How Self-Control Works, Why It Matters, and What You Can Do To Get More of It. Penguin Group.

Jones-Smith, Elise. (2016) Motivational Interviewing and the Stages of Change Theory, Theories of Counseling and Psychotherapy An Integrative Approach, chapter 10. Sage Publications Inc.

Maslow, Abraham. (1954) Motivation and Personality, New York;Harper.

Harris, K. B., & Miller, W. R. (1990) Behavioral self-control training for problem drinkers: Components of efficacy. Psychology of Addictive Behaviors, 4(2), 82–90.

Miller, W. R., Taylor, C. A., & West, J. C. (1980). Focused versus broad-spectrum behavior therapy for problem drinkers. Journal of Consulting and Clinical Psychology, 48(5), 590–601.

Miller, William & Rollnick, Stephen. (2013) Motivational Interviewing, Helping People Change, 3rd Edition, The Guilford Press.

Miller, W. (1983). Motivational Interviewing with Problem Drinkers. Behavioural Psychotherapy, 11(2), 147-172.

Moyers, Theresa. (2004) History and Happenstance: How Motivational Interviewing Got It's Start. Journal of Cognitive Psychotherapy: An International Quarterly, 18(4), 291- 298.

Peterson, Christopher. (2008) What Is Positive Psychology, and What Is It Not?. Psychology Today. 16 May.

Prochaska, J. O., & DiClemente, C. C. (1983) Stages and processes of self-change of smoking: Toward an integrative model of change. Journal of Consulting and Clinical Psychology, 51(3), 390–395.

Prochaska J. O, DiClemente CC, Norcross JC.(1992) In search of how people change. Applications to addictive behaviors. American Psychologist, Sep;47(9):1102-14.

Prochaska, James O., Norcross, James C. & DiClements, Carlos C. (2007) Changing for Good: A Revolutionary Six-Stage Program for

Overcoming Bad Habits and Moving Your Life Positively Forward, Harper Collins.

Prochaska, James O. and Velicer, Wayne F. (1997) The Transtheoretical Model of Health Behavior Change. American journal of health promotion 12(1) 38-48.

Seligman, Martin E.P. & Csikszentmilalyi, Mihaly. (2000) Positive Psychology:An Introduction. American Psychologist 55(1), 5-14.

Trepanowski, J.F., Bloomer, R.J. (2010) The impact of religious fasting on human health. Nutrition Journal 9, 57.

White, W. & Miller, W. (2007). The use of confrontation in addiction treatment: History, science and time for change. Counselor 8(4), 12-30.

Printed in Great Britain
by Amazon